MEALS THAT HEAL

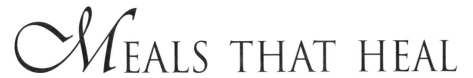

MEALS THAT HEAL

A Nutraceutical Approach to Diet and Health

LISA TURNER

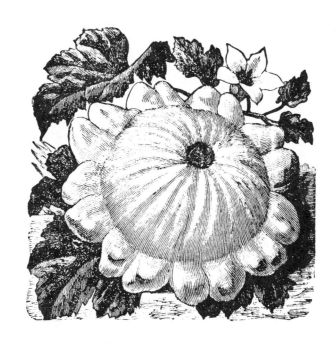

HEALING ARTS PRESS
ROCHESTER, VERMONT

Healing Arts Press
One Park Street
Rochester, Vermont 05767
www.gotoit.com

Note to the reader: This book is intended as an informational guide. The remedies, approaches, and techniques described herein are meant to supplement, and not to be a substitute for, professional medical care or treatment. They should not be used to treat a serious ailment without prior consultation with a qualified health care professional.

Library of Congress Cataloging-in-Publication Data

Turner, Lisa.
    Meals that heal : a nutraceutical approach to diet and health /
Lisa Turner.
       p.   cm.
    Includes bibliographical references and index.
    ISBN 0-89281-625-2
    1. Nutrition. 2. Diet therapy. I. Title.
RA784.T895   1996
613.2—dc20   96-21027
                                                           CIP

Printed and bound in the United States

10 9 8 7 6 5 4 3 2

Type design and layout by Peri Champine
This book was typeset in New Baskerville with Cochin and Vivante as the display typefaces

Healing Arts Press is a division of Inner Traditions International

Distributed to the book trade in Canada by Publishers Group West (PGW), Toronto, Ontario
Distributed to the health food trade in Canada by Alive Books, Toronto and Vancouver
Distributed to the book trade in the United Kingdom by Deep Books, London
Distributed to the book trade in Australia by Millennium Books, Newtown, N. S. W.
Distributed to the book trade in New Zealand by Tandem Press, Auckland
Distributed to the book trade in South Africa by Alternative Books, Ferndale

To my mother and father
for their endless generosity,
continuous support, and boundless love,
and to Alexandria—welcome to the world.

CONTENTS

Foreword   IX

Preface   X

Introduction   1

Part One

— ✐ —

THE FUNCTION OF FOOD

1 • Coming to Terms with Nutraceuticals   6
   Some Definitions • A Loaf of Bread, a Jug of Wine?

2 • The Changing of the Nutritional Guard   11
   The Making of a Movement: From "Less Is More" to "More Is More" •
   Aging Gracefully: The Search for Methuselah • Pioneers on New Frontiers

3 • The Best Defense: Whole Foods Versus Supplements   16
   The Times, They Sure Are Changing • No Magic Bullets

4 • Live Longer, Look Younger, Feel Better   23
   The Cancer Answer • Taking Heart: Cardiovascular Disease • Fighting Fat:
   Obesity and Hypertension • Living Stronger, Living Longer • The Fanfare
   about Free Radicals

5 • The Dynamic Dozen: The Twelve Best Places to Find Your Phytos   39
*Tomatoes • Cruciferous Vegetables • Soybeans • Whole Grains • Citrus Fruits •
Greens • Red/Orange/Yellow Fruits • Red/Orange/Yellow Vegetables • Fish •
Nuts and Seeds • Beans and Legumes • Onions and Garlic*

6 • The New Antioxidants and Novel Compounds   59
*Red Wine • Mushrooms • Ginger • Gamma Linolenic Acid (GLA) • Turmeric •
Green Tea • Bilberry • Green Foods • Ginkgo Biloba • Co-Q 10 • Conclusion*

Part Two

RECIPES

7 • A Few Notes on Preparation   82
Herbs and Other Substitutes • Cooking Beans and Legumes • Cooking Grains

8 • Tomatoes   86

9 • Cruciferous Vegetables   95

10 • Soybeans   104

11 • Grains   114

12 • Citrus Fruits   125

13 • Greens   134

14 • Red/Orange/Yellow Fruits   143

15 • Red/Orange/Yellow Vegetables   152

16 • Fish   160

17 • Nuts and Seeds   170

18 • Beans   179

19 • Onions and Garlic   190

Appendix: Finding Your Phytos   199

Notes   201

Bibliography   220

Index   223

FOREWORD

Not too long ago, the nutraceutical revolution began. This is very good news for all of us—better than most appreciate. Scientists and physicians have now joined together to conduct research to demonstrate more effectively the benefits of nutraceuticals—that is, foods or parts of foods that will prevent or ameliorate many of the afflictions that ail us and can aid not only in the prevention but also the treatment of disease. Garlic, for instance, contains compounds that show promise in retarding tumor growth. Whole grains, vegetable oil, and nuts contain vitamin E, which has been shown to significantly slow cardiovascular disease. Peppermint, ginger, and fennel seeds help folks with indigestion and stomach distress. The nutraceutical list is long.

Most people still don't know exactly what nutraceuticals are, but as the media continue to dole out bits and pieces of information on the healing power of carrots and cucumbers, consumers are ravenous for more information. Countless articles have been written on nutraceuticals, designer foods, and phytochemicals, but no one has written a comprehensive book geared toward the consumer, until now. *Meals That Heal* is a lucid and inclusive text that clearly explains nutraceuticals and their role in health and longevity.

Let's not fool ourselves. Many of the diets that we eat and the dietary supplements that we take, although highly promising, need to be medically evaluated to definitely prove whether they help us or not. Ongoing and future research will attempt to identify areas of specific benefit. My crystal ball says that we'll all be pleasantly surprised in the very near future.

But what do we do in the meanwhile? Abundant information presently exists that clearly indicates that it is worthwhile—now—to eat certain diets and take certain dietary supplements. In this fine book, Lisa Turner presents rationally based guidelines on how to make such judgments. We live in a period of nutrababble where much confusion abounds, leaving all of us with difficult and often frustrating choices. *Meals That Heal* will help us make the proper decisions.

Stephen L. DeFelice, M.D.
Chairman, The Foundation for Innovation in Medicine

PREFACE

When I began to write this book, I was working for a nutraceuticals company involved in developing concentrated and standardized food-based supplements. In other words, their goal was to identify certain active ingredients that had proven health benefits and extract them from food, to be used in pill, powder, tablet, or liquid forms for the greatest health benefit. It was a compelling concept, and one that more than a few companies have attempted.

At that time, I saw—and still do see—the value of concentrated nutraceutical formulas. But during my stint at that company, I noticed a certain wariness on the part of some members of the natural-products industry about the wisdom of extracting compounds from food, isolating them into pill form, and hoping for the same efficacy that nature provides in its infinite and innate wisdom. How could vitamin companies hope to compete with the elegant and efficient packaging of Mother Nature? I also watched the definitions and dynamics of the concept of "nutraceuticals" evolving at a dizzying pace. Did it include fortified bread and milk with calcium added? Or was the field limited to novel and exotic compounds that no one can find on his or her grocer's shelves?

These were questions that no one seemed equipped to answer. So I gave up on the term nutraceuticals and began searching for a more comprehensive definition, one with some clarity—and sanity. One definition emerged immediately: nutraceuticals as vitamins, supplements, and extracts are largely derived from *phytochemicals* in plant foods and *zoochemicals* in animal-based sources of nutrition, compounds that have specific health benefits. Because the focus of this book is on plant sources of healing compounds, I generally use the term "phytochemicals"; "phyto" refers exclusively to plants. The term "zoochemicals" was coined by Anthony Almada—a nutritional biochemist at Myogenix in Palo Alto, California—to describe healthful compounds in animal products, including fish, eggs, dairy products, and meat.

No one in the field of so-called nutraceuticals seemed to be paying much attention to the idea of food itself, and food combinations, in healing regimens. Instead, vitamin and supplement manufacturers were dizzy with the prospects of capturing and isolating these ill-researched compounds and stuffing them into tablets and capsules. It's a seductive idea, but the danger is the loss of perspective—that is, these compounds came from *food* in the first place. The concept of well-balanced meals with a sensible and sane supplement program was increasingly ignored as scientists continued to focus only on individual compounds, not seeing the forest for the phytochemical trees.

The world of nutraceuticals thus seemed a wildly spinning planet in a universe of concentrated herbal extracts with unwieldy scientific names that few people can even pronounce, let alone find at the local grocery. Ego-gratifying terms like "glutathione-S-transferase" and "epigallocatechin gallate" were often used erroneously and unnecessarily. Stephen L. DeFelice, M.D.—chairman of the Foundation for Innovation in Medicine in Cranford, New Jersey, and the man who coined the term nutraceuticals in the first place—says simply, "It's all become nothing more than a bunch of nutrababble."

I could see the need for a comprehensive, clear, and user-friendly book on the value of phytochemicals and zoochemicals in food forms, the concept of meals that can heal, and the specific functions of whole foods. Hence the term I use in this text: functional foods. It's far from perfect—aren't all foods functional, in one way or another, be it through exquisite nutritional value or sheer gustatory satisfaction? But it's the closest any term in the field comes to expressing what I want to relay.

So as we take a tour through this brave new world of functional foods, here's what you can expect: some definitions of various terms you'll come to hear on a near-daily basis, a history of how the whole movement started, a description of categories of various phytochemicals and some zoochemicals (for those of you who thrive on scientific nomenclature and sixteen-syllable words), and an enumeration of the most valid studies I could find showing the value of phytochemicals and in some cases zoochemicals. (I have attempted to use human research wherever possible, but in some cases, only animal studies are available.) You'll also find out which foods you can use in your daily life to enhance your overall health, specific benefits of those foods, a list of the top twelve foods in terms of their phytochemical density, and 120 recipe suggestions using those top twelve foods.

Additionally, you'll notice an intense focus on antioxidants, since these are the compounds on which the most comprehensive and valid scientific studies have been conducted to date. I've also included a section on "novel" antioxidants and healing compounds—the up-and-coming contenders in the world of nutrition that are the subjects of noted and compelling research. And while I primarily encourage and promote the use of foods in their whole form, the existence of hundreds of solid scientific studies regarding the health benefits of supplement use makes it impossible for me to condone a diet consisting of whole foods alone. So I've attempted to define a middle ground, in which diet is the main source of nutrition, with supplements providing extra protection.

And now for the fun part of the trip: since the focus of this book *is* on meals that heal, this text incorporates discussions of real foods that can help prevent and even heal disease, including more than 100 recipes using the biggest and best of the healing foods. That's the itinerary. Sit back, relax, and enjoy the ride.

∽

My deepest appreciation to Robin and all the talented folks at Inner Traditions for their endless patience and wisdom; to Steve Petusevsky for tasting, testing, and reviewing recipes; to Marcia and Jon Zimmerman for helping to clear the muddy waters of phytochemical classification; and to Anthony Almada, for sharing with me his overwhelming knowledge and giving me the gift of his time and patience.

My most fervent thanks to the many people who have helped me with this book including Dr. Stephen DeFelice at the Foundation for Innovation in Medicine, Jethren Phillips and Neil Blomquist of Spectrum Naturals, Frank Ford and Jon Goodman of Arrowhead Mills, Brady Whitlow of Muir Glen, Ken Vickerstaff of White Wave, George Larsen of GCI Nutrients, Chuck Brice and Rod Ausich of Kemin Industries, and Sabinsa Corporation for their research and support; Dr. Phil Taylor at the National Cancer Institute; Dr. Paul LaChance of Rutgers University; Dr. Dexter Morris at the University of North Carolina School of Medicine; Lenore Kohlmeier, Ph.D., at the University of North Carolina School of Medicine; Odyssey Nutriceutical Sciences; the National Cancer Institute; the American Heart Association; and all the many other generous and patient individuals who gave me their time during interviews and shared with me their knowledge.

INTRODUCTION

Over the last few years, a barrage of information regarding the healing properties of food has come into the public light. We've known for years that vitamin C prevents scurvy, B vitamins prevent beriberi, and calcium helps build strong bones. But recent discoveries of certain agents in foods that can help prevent—or even heal—disease are ushering in a new and exciting paradigm, changing forever the way we look at foods and inaugurating the concept of creating meals that heal.

Garlic, for instance, contains organosulfur compounds that have been shown to reduce blood pressure, lower cholesterol levels, and reduce blood clotting. Broccoli contains substances called sulforaphane and indoles that may help prevent cancer. And soybeans contain phytic acid and protease inhibitors, which have been shown to be helpful in lowering cholesterol levels and warding off cancer. These substances, called phytochemicals, and the foods that contain them can be collectively lumped under the terms "nutraceuticals" or "functional foods"—that is, foods that can help to prevent and cure disease.

As of this writing, no one has been able to agree on the divisions and definitions for these nutrient compounds—in fact, no one has been able to even agree upon the spelling of the word "nutraceuticals" (some spell it "nutriceuticals"). But one point upon which most experts agree is that nutrition in the '90s is a radically different field. Scientists are sailing uncharted waters, in an attempt to discover and colonize territories of nutrition for the millennium.

Even the U.S. Food and Drug Administration (FDA) has finally, if somewhat grudgingly, acknowledged the fact that foods can heal. One FDA expert defined phytochemicals as "substances found in edible fruits and vegetables that may be ingested by humans daily in gram quantities, and that exhibit a potential for modulating human metabolism in a manner favorable for cancer prevention." The agency has recognized the connection between nutrition and potential causes and cures of disease, especially in the following areas:[1]

- Antioxidant vitamins and cancer
- Calcium and osteoporosis
- Sodium and hypertension
- Dietary fats and cardiovascular disease
- Dietary fats and cancer
- Fiber and cardiovascular disease
- Zinc and immune function

The facts and figures relating diet to disease prevention are no longer the province of unwieldy scientific texts or bodies of arcane research, and the concept of functional foods is no longer solely in the realm of scientific and medical journals. A 1995 issue of *Newsweek* featured a cover story on functional foods, extolling the virtues of phytochemicals in foods and exposing a huge consumer market to the concepts and language of phytochemicals and functional foods. Countless newsletters and magazines across the United States have taken up the topic of functional foods, and articles about foods that heal fill the lifestyle pages of leading newspapers nationwide. And what the research and the researchers are coming to recognize is that Mom was right after all. If you want to be healthy, eat your fruits and vegetables. And garlic, and soybeans.

It may seem too good to be true. Can a regular diet of tomatoes and cruciferous vegetables ward off cancer and heart disease? Can meals really heal? More and more studies are sounding an unequivocal "yes" to this question, but getting accurate, easy-to-understand information on the *proven* health benefits of certain foods is a Herculean task at times. Hence the mission of this book: to discuss functional foods, phytochemicals, and zoochemicals and their proven health benefits; to examine different types of healing substances in foods; and to offer recipes that use these healing foods to make healthy and delicious meals.

What this book will *not* attempt to do is to discuss the health benefits of dozens of different vitamins, herbs, and other supplements. Hundreds of comprehensive books on the benefits of vitamins, minerals, and fiber are on the market today. For that reason, we focus on three main areas: the vitamins (A, C, and E), novel antioxidants, and other phytochemicals and zoochemicals in foods that have specific and proven health benefits. Additionally, because whole foods are such an important consideration, we focus on finding phytochemicals in your refrigerator, rather than on the supplement shelves, with a brief exploration of both sides of the whole-foods-versus-supplements discussion.

Another point: the American focus has recently been toward "less"—less salt, less fat, less cholesterol, less calories, less food choices—often, sadly enough, to the exclusion of the concept of "more"—that is, more vegetables, more fiber, more whole foods and grains. In this "more," the expansion of our palates and plates, we will find the healing substances in foods that may have eluded many of us until now.

PART ONE

THE FUNCTION OF FOOD

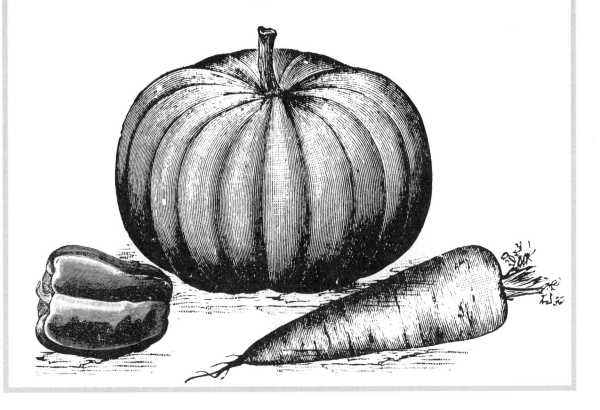

1

COMING TO TERMS WITH NUTRACEUTICALS

In the emerging and rapidly evolving field of nutritional healing, the nomenclature is often unavoidably esoteric, and the categories of "nutraceuticals," "functional foods," and "designer foods" are not as neat and tidy as we would perhaps like. We might settle for saying that functional foods are foods that contain substances with specific, proven healing benefits. In theory, using this broad definition, we could include everything from Wheat Chex to fiber-packed, vitamin-fortified energy bars. Our focus, however, is on whole, unaltered foods that contain phytochemicals and zoochemicals—those specific compounds that are believed to help increase life span, prevent illness, and even cure diseases—as well as other, more familiar dietary components, such as essential fatty acids, fiber, and the antioxidant vitamins A, C, and E.

SOME DEFINITIONS

Grappling with the nomenclature in vogue is a sticky but unavoidable task. The two terms currently fighting for the limelight, and often used interchangeably, are "nutraceuticals" and "functional foods," with "nutraceuticals" a nose ahead in the race. Since the term "nutraceuticals" is frequently used in an impossibly broad sense to describe a wide range of different theories, products, and disciplines, let's settle on a few more definitions:

- *Nutraceuticals* are concentrated products, often in supplement form, with a standardized dosage and a proven level of efficacy in the prevention and/or treatment of disease. They may include nutritional products designed to enhance performance, to encourage weight loss, to treat minor maladies such as insomnia and fatigue, or to treat more serious conditions such as cardiovascular disease and cancer.

- *Phytochemicals* are substances that occur naturally in plants and that have the ability to prevent or cure disease.
- *Zoochemicals* are substances that occur naturally in animal products and that may prevent or cure disease.
- *Functional foods* are foods that offer proven health benefits and medicinal properties—for instance, garlic and green tea—and contain phytochemicals in their unadulterated states.
- *Designer foods* include bioengineered foods and genetically manipulated foodstuffs, as well as fortified foods, which can range from bread with added B vitamins to fruit juices enriched with carotenoids.

The concept of nutraceuticals is seductive, but elusive. The field is changing rapidly and dramatically, and many conflicting notions and views—as well as research findings—spring up every day. One common reality emerges immediately: most of us don't have carefully labeled bottles of triterpenes and polyphenols lined up on our kitchen shelves. Most of us do, however, have refrigerators filled with broccoli and carrots and cupboards stocked with grains and beans.

Michael Goodman, director of research publications at Decision Resources, a consulting firm in life sciences in Waltham, Massachusetts, points out, "The vitamin industry is starting to take off in the field of nutraceuticals, but things aren't going to happen real fast. There's an enormous amount of science that still has to happen. Consumers like to think of food as food, something that fills your tummy and makes you feel good, and the association with nutraceuticals and pharmaceuticals may put them off. You won't see food companies launching nutraceutical TV dinners. It just ain't gonna happen. And even though nutraceuticals are a growing trend, there's not going to be an aisle in the grocery store devoted to them."

The U.S. government has yet to acknowledge or establish a definition for functional foods, but other countries are actively researching and advocating the use of foods in disease prevention. Germany and Japan are the leading countries in promoting functional foods, peddling everything from phytochemical-fortified cookies to sodas laced with vitamins. The Japanese Ministry of Health and Welfare has instituted an eloquent working model. Foods for specified health use and disease prevention are defined by the health ministry as functional foods and include substances that enhance

FOOD STUFFS

Only a few decades ago, researchers established a standard definition for bioactive substances in food, determining the caloric value and differentiating between fat, protein, and carbohydrates. Since then, a number of generally recognized components of food have been identified:

- Micronutrients, such as vitamins and minerals.
- Macronutrients, such as fats, proteins, and carbohydrates, which provide calories or energy.
- Fiber.
- Conditionally essential nutrients or orthomolecular components, such as co-Q 10, that are produced by the body and may be needed by some individuals in greater amounts, depending on genetic predisposition or environmental factors.
- Phytonutrients, or phytochemicals—that is, compounds that are not produced in the human body, but are available in plants.
- Zoonutrients, or zoochemicals—compounds generally not produced by the body, or produced in small, often inadequate amounts, and found in animal products.

∽

immune function, aid in the prevention of diseases such as hypertension and diabetes, and help slow the aging process.[1]

It's really not too good to be true.

A LOAF OF BREAD, A JUG OF WINE?

Back in the good old days—say, 1988—it used to be simpler. Food was the stuff you put on a plate, set on a placemat, and flanked with fork and spoon. It was the stuff you salted and peppered and chewed and swallowed. It was the stuff you shared with friends and family, because it tasted good and was somehow good for you. Now, while sometimes—in spite of Freudian ideas to the contrary—a cigar is just a cigar, a carrot is much, much more.

What exactly is food? Broadly defined, it is any of the many substances that keep you alive. As early as the beginning of this century, scientists were already beginning to isolate and identify trace constituents of food, finding that they contained substances, including amino acids, that could prevent disease. These compounds were named "vitamins," from the Latin meaning "life-giving amines or amino acids." Thus began the first step on the long road toward recognition of food substances and health.

Today, new compounds and classes of phytochemicals are being discovered on a weekly basis. In general, phytochemicals—those compounds in foods that may offer health benefits and make us live longer, look younger, and feel better—are grouped on the basis of the similarities of their protective functions. Much or most of the focus has been on the basis of the antioxidant value of phytochemicals. We take an in-depth look at antioxidants in chapter 6, but for now we can briefly define antioxidants as beneficial compounds that quench the activity of cell-damaging free radicals—unstable, reactive, and often harmful chemicals formed in the body through normal metabolic processes and from external toxins, such as cigarette smoke or air pollution. Let's glance at some of the most important types of phytochemicals, the ones that seem to come up over and over again as we talk about healing foods.

Carotenoids

The humble carrot has risen of late to a status near sublime, as scientists continue to extol the virtues of foods containing carotenoids. Carotenoids are identifiable in foods by their characteristic red, orange, or yellow color—think of carrots, tomatoes, oranges, and so forth. They're also present in greens, parsley, and various other fruits and vegetables.

The phytochemicals in this class act as potent antioxidants. Estimates number more than 600 naturally occurring carotenoids; of these, about 5 to

10 percent act as what are called "vitamin A precursors"—that is, they are transformed in the body into vitamin A—including alpha-carotene, epsilon-carotene, and the current darling of the nutrition scene, beta-carotene. These nutritional dynamos have been associated with protection against various cancers, including lung, colon, breast, uterine, and prostate cancers, and they enhance immune response.[2]

Beta-carotene is perhaps the most widely and substantively researched of the carotenoids. Numerous epidemiological studies demonstrate that this valuable antioxidant can protect against cancer and stroke, help prevent cardiovascular disease, enhance immune function, lower cholesterol levels, and help prevent cataracts. Researchers at the National Cancer Institute (NCI) have recognized the health benefits of beta-carotene and its role in reducing the risk of cancer. Beta-carotene is also one of the most readily available antioxidants from food sources; it occurs naturally in a variety of red and orange fruits and vegetables, ranging from mangos and papayas to carrots and pumpkins.

Limonoids

As reflected in their name, limonoids are found primarily in the rinds of citrus fruits such as lemons, grapefruit, and oranges. Limonoids are a subclass of the broader class of phytochemicals called terpenes; they appear to be most beneficial in relation to lung disease and may also be valuable in preventing cancer because they stimulate the production of enzymes that can help deactivate carcinogens. Research indicates that D-limonene helps protect against cancer by detoxifying carcinogens in the liver. Lemons, limes, oranges, tangerines, grapefruit, and other citrus fruits contain monoterpenes, which can help prevent cancer and inhibit changes in already malignant cells.[3] You can easily incorporate limonoids into your diet—try the Red Grapefruit Ambrosia or the Citrus Salad with Spiced Raisins in the recipe section.

Sulfur compounds

These powerful anticarcinogens also have antibacterial and antifungal properties. Found in onions, garlic, scallions, leeks, radishes, and mustard, sulfur compounds and their related constituents—including thiols, allylic sulfides, and isothiocyanates—help reduce the risk of cancer, lower cholesterol levels, decrease blood clotting, have antibacterial and antifungal properties, and show potent antioxidant effects. They're easy to add to your diet—just toss a handful of chopped onion into soups and stir-fries or season your food with a little extra garlic. And try the Leek and Morel Sauté or the Baked Garlic Cloves with Toasted Pita in the recipe section.

A PHYTOCHEMICAL WHO'S WHO

The list of phytochemicals in foods is daunting and not relevant to our daily lives unless we become well versed in nutrition and cellular molecular biology. It is, however, worthwhile to identify some of the key ingredients in this endlessly simmering cauldron of nutra-soup. Following is a list of the main categories of phytochemicals and some of their subcategories.

ORGANOSULFUR COMPOUNDS
Allylic sulfides, sulforaphane, isothiocyanates

CAROTENOIDS
Alpha-carotene, beta-carotene, lutein, lycopene, zeaxanthin, cryptoxanthin, canthaxanthin

PHENOLS
Catechins, polyphenol catechins, ellagic acid, glycyrrhizin

FLAVONOIDS
Genistein, quercetin

TERPENOIDS
D-Limonene

INDOLES
Indole-3-carbinol

ORGANIC ACIDS
Phytic acid, phenolic acid

ISOPRENOIDS
Vitamin E/tocopherols, co-Q 10, tocotrienols

RETINOIDS
Vitamin A

ASCORBIC ACID
Vitamin C

EFAS
Omega-3 fatty acids, omega-6 fatty acids

FIBER
Hemicellulose, cellulose, lignins, pectins

Sources: Marcia Zimmerman & Associates, Westlake Village, CA; Anthony Almada, Myogenix, Palo Alto, CA

Genistein

The unassuming little soybean has taken on heroic properties in the face of recent research that shows that genistein, found in a variety of soy products including tofu, tempeh, and soy milk, may not only prevent cancer and help inhibit tumor growth, but may also cause cancer cells to transform into normal cells. If soy isn't now a regular part of your diet, try the Coconut-Soy Cakes or Tempeh with Garlic Sauce listed in the recipe section.

Indoles

Found in cabbage, broccoli, brussels sprouts, and many greens, indoles have been shown to detoxify carcinogens and may reduce the risk of breast cancer and other cancers. You can easily incorporate cruciferous vegetables and greens into your diet as side dishes or as colorful additions to soups and salads. Or try the Broccoli-Pine Nut Casserole and the Creamy Spinach Soup in the recipe section.

These few examples illustrate the powerful disease-prevention potential of foods. A comprehensive list of phytochemical compounds would include thousands and thousands of substances and constituents.

All plant foods—or almost all plant foods—have some kind of beneficial phytochemical effect. Therein lies the problem with classifications. No one seems to agree on categories and subcategories or on the definitions of beneficial and nonbeneficial. Numerous other phytochemicals exist in the foods we eat every day. In chapter 5, we discuss twelve of the most nutritionally dense foods in terms of phytochemical and zoochemical content—the dynamic dozen—the foods upon which the recipes in this book are based.

2

THE CHANGING OF
THE NUTRITIONAL GUARD

THE MAKING OF A MOVEMENT:
FROM "LESS IS MORE" TO "MORE IS MORE"

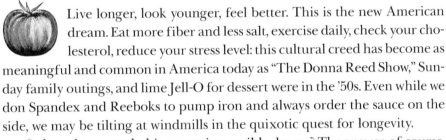Live longer, look younger, feel better. This is the new American dream. Eat more fiber and less salt, exercise daily, check your cholesterol, reduce your stress level: this cultural creed has become as meaningful and common in America today as "The Donna Reed Show," Sunday family outings, and lime Jell-O for dessert were in the '50s. Even while we don Spandex and Reeboks to pump iron and always order the sauce on the side, we may be tilting at windmills in the quixotic quest for longevity.

So how do we reach this not-so-impossible dream? The answer, of course, is that we keep on exercising regularly, stressing out infrequently, and revising our diet. But herein lies the elusive question: *what*, exactly, do we need to revise?

The last 20 years have ushered in what we might call the changing of the nutritional guard: that is, the recognition of food as nutrient dense and health enhancing and a movement away from less is more to *more* is more. Hippocrates said "Let your food be your medicine; let your medicine be your food." For tens of thousands of years, human beings subsisted on a balanced diet of vegetables, grains, fruits, nuts, and so forth. The diet of most of our ancestors 20,000 years ago was about 75 percent from plant sources—including leaves, seeds, fruits, and tubers—with the remaining 25 percent from animal products. People didn't monitor their fat intake or tally up grams of fiber in their diets. And for years, the American public ate in much the same way—blissfully unaware of fiber and cholesterol, with an ease and simplicity lacking today—some vegetables, some grains, some meat. It wasn't the superlative regimen, but it was easy enough.

Over the years, guilt replaced gustatory pleasures as worried Americans found themselves getting more heavy and less healthy. Hollandaise sauce became a fragile memory as newly health- and weight-conscious Americans took over the reins of the nutrition cart. From their constant calorie and cholesterol counting sprung forth the notion of less is more. Less fat, less salt, less animal protein. And while these are in many regards admirable goals, one point was sadly overlooked. In the fervor to reduce and remove certain unhealthy elements of the national diet, few people considered the possibility that we might actually need *more*: more vegetables, more fruits, more nutrition in general.

The recognition of food as a means of healing isn't a new concept in most cultures. In the United States, the nutritive value of food was officially circumscribed in the mid-1950s, when the U.S. government introduced the "four food groups" concept. Erroneous and incomplete though some of those government guidelines may have been, federal dietary recommendations set the stage for further awareness and growth in the meals-can-heal movement.

Nutrition as an earnest practice gained a strong and irrevocable foothold in the early 1960s, when vegetarianism began to grow in popularity, championed by a nascent back-to-the-earth movement and bolstered by the introduction of macrobiotics and various healing practices from other cultures. In the mid '60s, diet was elevated to a status of pseudo-religion, fed by environmental fears over pesticides and preservatives, moral dilemmas, and health concerns and further fueled by a near-fanatic cult fervor. Meat was eschewed by those in the nutritional know, and tofu became the gustatory drug of choice for a growing number of health-conscious Americans.

The nutrition movement continued through the trend-conscious '70s and body-conscious '80s, as the general public became acutely aware of a growing body of research linking diet to disease. In the mid-1980s, researchers began seriously to explore the role of nutrition and food, studying such ingredients as calcium and fiber and focusing on evidence that deficiencies or inadequacies of certain nutrients often resulted in increased incidence of disease or dysfunction. This drastic scientific shift from a focus on nutrients as substances to treat specific diseases caused by nutritional deficiencies—such as vitamin C deficiency and scurvy or thiamin deficiency and beriberi—ushered in the new nutrition of the '90s.

Nutrition and diet have been elevated to a noble status, wherein the focus is no longer on maintaining the marginal amount of nutrition needed to sustain life, but rather on pursuing a well-defined system for optimal health and longevity. Most Americans aren't worried about scurvy (or beriberi or rickets, for that matter). Now we fret about heart disease, cancer, obesity, and other major maladies. And nutritionists and researchers alike have finally acknowledged the intimate connection between diet and life-threatening diseases. Other conditions, including gastrointestinal disorders, impaired immune function, and kidney disease, are thought by numerous researchers to have a nutritional link.

Slowly the focus began to shift from the "less is more" religion of the '80s to the "more is more" approach of the '90s, with increasing research on fortified, supplemented, and—in some cases—genetically engineered foods. This current mode of thought is so strong that in the early '90s the NCI initiated a five-year, $20 million project to study experimental processed and supplemented foods fortified with natural anticarcinogenic ingredients, such as garlic extract, licorice extract, and soybean meal.[1]

AGING GRACEFULLY: THE SEARCH FOR METHUSELAH

Another fundamental paradigm shift occurred when researchers introduced a radical, yet elegantly simple, concept: the difference between *health* span and *life* span. As interest in gerontology and the mechanisms of aging increased in the scientific community, researchers began to acknowledge the fact that humans cannot expect to radically extend our average life expectancy by more than a few years. That's the bad news. The good news is that we may be able to radically increase our health span—that is, we can reasonably expect to extend the number of years we live healthy, fruitful lives, and reduce age-related disease and disability.

Over the past few decades, the American life span has increased to 78.5 years for women and 71.75 for men—a 53 percent increase since the turn of the century. But how many of those added years are spent in health and overall vitality? Historically, degenerative disease begins to manifest in varying degrees anywhere between the ages of 45 and 60. The goal of researchers now is to retard those age-related diseases, with the potential promise of offering the population in general the assurance of extended health well into the later years of life. And the answers they are finding focus on preventive care—mainly, through proper nutrition.

"The concept of health span is elegant but simple, and is congruent with the concept of wellness and prevention," says Michael Osband, M.D., chief of

Further gains in life expectancy will occur, but these gains will be modest. However, it is not clear whether a longer life implies better health [or] a prolonged period of frailty and dependency.

Olshanskey et al., *Science*[2]

the Division of Pediatric Hematology-Oncology, Boston City Hospital and Boston University School of Medicine. "Historically, humans were probably genetically programmed to live for only 40 years. . . . In fact, in 1900, health span—that portion of life span during which most people are generally healthy—was the same as life span, about 40 years."

Since then, says Osband—who also runs a Cambridge-based firm called Odyssey Nutriceutical Sciences—advances in public health, sanitation, antibiotics, nutrition, and overall medical knowledge have extended life span to nearly 80 years. "But we have not done nearly so well at extending health span, which has remained at the genetically predetermined 40 years," he says. "After that time, there is a progressive loss of wellness and function, and a dramatic increase in the incidence of age-related disease, examples of which include cardiovascular disease, neurological degeneration, arthritis, cancer, infectious disease, cataracts, and osteoporosis. The clinical goal of functional foods and nutraceuticals is to prolong health span until it is equal or nearly equal to life span."

Major causes of death—cancer, stroke, heart disease, and obesity and hypertension—have been linked to diet through reams of solid scientific research. Now the focus is on other types of degenerative, age-related disorders: adult-onset diabetes, cataracts, motorneuron diseases, and possibly Alzheimer's. Other research indicates that cognitive function and central nervous system activity are related to diet and nutrition. Additionally, blood-antioxidant concentrations, particularly of vitamins C and E and beta-carotene, are related to aging, and improved antioxidant status in the body may significantly impact many disorders associated with aging.[3]

PIONEERS ON NEW FRONTIERS

As we've said, the idea of foods as healing isn't a new concept. For thousands of years, various civilizations have used foods and herbs for healing. Garlic has been used for medicinal purposes for centuries in Egypt, Rome, Greece, India, and numerous other cultures. It is said that the builders of the pyramids ate large amounts of garlic to maintain their strength for that formidable task. Ginger was used extensively to treat nausea, fever, and whooping cough in China and Japan for thousands of years, and yogurt was widely prescribed in India as a cure for bowel and stomach ailments. All of these societies intuitively recognized the intrinsic value of food in the role of health, and years of empirical research confirmed the positive effects.

But Americans in the late 20th century have demanded more than experimental and speculative documentation. The call for substantive, scientific research on foods and healing grew louder, but what exactly was the scientific community attempting to find and define? Nutritionists and re-searchers grappled for years with the arduous task of categorizing foods with healing properties.

The first attempt at classifying this unwieldy topic came from DeFelice, who coined the term "nutraceuticals" (note the original spelling) along with a reasonably comprehensive but admittedly broad definition: "Any substance that may be considered a food or part of a food and provides medical or health benefits, including the prevention and treatment of disease. Such products may range from dietary supplements, diets, and isolated nutrients to genetically engineered 'designer' foods and processed foods such as cereals, soups, and beverages."

DeFelice's attempts at defining healing foods was borne from his frustration at the scientific community's insufficient attempts to classify these substances and from the inadequate definition of food itself. "You cannot define the difference between a food and a drug," he says. "The Food and Drug Administration defines it legally: food is something you eat, but once you make a claim that it works medically, it becomes a drug. What we have now are dietary supplements, brews, teas, extracts—all with claims for medical benefits. Are these foods?"[4]

Perhaps the one event that changed the face of the phytochemical world was what DeFelice calls the "calcium-fiber-fish oil" revolution in the early 1980s. Because of the extensive amount of scientific research regarding these three substances, in journals ranging from the *New England Journal of Medicine* to the *Journal of the American Medical Association*, the medical community finally, if somewhat grudgingly, threw in the towel and their scrub suits and joined the legions of nutrition devotees. Numerous physicians began not only to prescribe these products to their patients, but also to use them (if sometimes furtively) themselves.

From there, it was only a few short steps to the notion that green tea can prevent cancer and that carrots and broccoli can act as powerful antioxidants. A steady and growing amount of research began to accumulate during the late '80s on the uses of beta-carotene to fight lung cancer, vitamin E to prevent heart disease, fiber to lower cholesterol, and numerous other phytochemicals.

As physicians began cautiously to extol the virtues of vitamins and whole foods, their patients began to listen and to demand more information. By the mid-1990s, reams of research in superb scientific journals had firmly established the role of countless phytochemicals in foods and their effects on health. And as we enter the new millennium, it's probably safe to say that the world of nutrition will never be the same.

3

THE BEST DEFENSE
Whole Foods Versus Supplements

It would be seductive indeed to claim that we can get all of our nutritional necessities from whole foods. Unfortunately, this may not be the case. Because most Americans don't eat the right kinds of food, it's a tenuous bet at best that the average daily diet will provide adequate nutrition to ward off disease and even minor maladies. Most of the research that's been done on phytochemicals, particularly the antioxidants, has been with therapeutic doses—that is, doses that are high enough to prevent or even cure disease.

While our daily diets may contain enough vitamin C to prevent scurvy or vitamin B to hold beriberi at bay, the nutritional lineup of the average American diet is generally ill equipped to provide substantial protection against chronic degenerative disease. On a more practical level, in many cases we simply can't eat enough food to acquire the therapeutic doses that have been shown to prevent disease. For example, numerous studies demonstrate that vitamin E provides substantial health benefits and prevention of disease at levels ranging from 400 to 1,000 IU per day. At the low end, that translates into approximately 53 cups of wheat-germ oil or 200 avocados. Even if we were, by some robust feat, able to achieve this ridiculous level of food consumption, the fat content of such a diet would grossly offset any nutritional benefits realized by an increased level of vitamin E.

Which is certainly not to say that we can live by pills alone. Food is complex, and it contains a multitude of substances, some not yet fully understood or identified, that may work in concert with each other. Consequently, it would be an egregious error to assume that so long as we gulp down a handful of pills with every meal, we can satisfy our nutritional needs on a diet of French fries and rum-raisin ice cream.

So what's the verdict: whole foods or pills? The answer, according to most experts, is both.

The Times, They Sure Are Changing

Every day, the lifestyle section of most major newspapers offers at least one article on the benefits of a whole-foods diet, extolling the virtues of more cruciferous vegetables and waxing poetic about the humble legume. Health experts also continue to recommend that we consume diets based on whole foods and that we dramatically increase our consumption of vegetables, fruits, and whole grains.

This widespread media coverage, backed up by ardent promotion from nutritionists and health-care specialists, has finally captured the attention—and shopping lists and pocketbooks—of most Americans. More than 60 percent of Americans now say they believe there is a connection between food and mood, and 75 percent say they recognize the connection between diet and longevity.[1]

In a 1994 survey sponsored by Thomas Food Industry Register and Find/SVP in New York, 94 percent of shoppers said they had changed their eating habits to create healthier diets. Americans seem increasingly to be buying fruits and vegetables more for their nutritional benefit and less out of habit: when asked about their reasons for purchasing fresh vegetables, 57 percent of women and 37 percent of men were interested in beta-carotene, 34 percent of women and 25 percent of men were looking for vitamin C, and 33 percent of women and 17 percent of men were interested in vitamin A. Additionally, 41 percent of women and 19 percent of men said they were concerned about cancer prevention.

The most compelling argument for disease prevention based on diet—rather than supplements—is that whole food contains as-yet-unidentified compounds that can magnify the effects of identified phytochemicals. Foods in general contain a multitude of phytochemical and other compounds, the effects of which are not fully understood. Additionally, a growing body of research from laboratory and human studies is suggesting that phytochemicals work best in concert. Most of the main cancer-fighting ingredients in fruits and vegetables, especially antioxidants, are most effective in combination with each other, and a mixture of a variety of plant nutrients can help increase the efficacy of certain cancer drugs.

No Magic Bullets

Beta-carotene, perhaps the best-known antioxidant, has been widely acclaimed as a sort of magic bullet, the prom queen of the phytochemicals. Some researchers, however, point out that it might not be beta-carotene that's offering superlative health benefits, but rather some of its relatives in the carotenoid family, or other phytochemical compounds altogether. As Philip Taylor, M.D., Scientific Director of the Cancer Prevention Studies Branch of the NCI says, "It may be that we've crowned the wrong queen."

Table 1

SOURCES OF CAROTENOIDS

MICROGRAMS PER OUNCE

Food	Beta-carotene	Alpha-carotene	Lutein and Zeaxanthin	Lycopene	Crypto-xanthin
Apricot, dried	4,990	0	0	245	0
Asparagus	127	3	181	0	0
Avocado	10	0	91	0	0
Beet greens	726	1	2,183	0	0
Broccoli	369	0	510	0	0
Brussels sprouts	136	2	369	0	0
Cabbage	61	0	238	0	0
Cantaloupe	851	10	0	0	0
Carrot	2,240	1,049	74	0	0
Celery	201	0	1,021	0	0
Chicory	972	0	2,920	0	0
Corn	14	14	221	0	0
Dill	1,276	0	1,899	0	0
Endive	369	0	1,134	0	0
Fennel	1,259	0	0	0	0
Grapefruit, pink	371	0	0	953	0
Greens, collard	1,531	0	4,621	0	0
Greens, mustard	765	0	2,807	0	0
Guava juice	77	7	0	947	0
Kale	1,332	0	6,209	0	0
Kiwi	0	0	223	0	0

Food	Beta-carotene	Alpha-carotene	Lutein and Zeaxanthin	Lycopene	Crypto-xanthin
Leeks	284	0	539	0	0
Romaine	539	0	1,616	0	0
Mango	369	0	0	0	15
Nectarine	29	0	4	0	12
Okra	48	8	1,928	0	0
Parsley	1,503	0	2,892	0	0
Peach, dried	2,624	0	53	0	71
Peas, green	99	5	482	0	0
Pepper, green	65	3	198	0	0
Pepper, red	624	17	1,928	0	0
Pepper, yellow	43	26	218	0	0
Plum	122	0	68	0	0
Pumpkin	879	1077	425	0	0
Scallion	241	0	0	595	0
Spinach	1,559	0	3,572	0	0
Squash, summer	119	3	340	0	0
Squash, winter	680	3	1	0	0
Sweet potato	2,495	0	0	0	0
Swiss chard	1,034	13	3,119	0	0
Tomato juice	255	0	94	2,432	0
Tomato paste	482	0	54	1,843	0
Tomato, raw	147	0	28	879	0
Watermelon	65	0.3	4	1,162	0
Watercress	1,177	0	3,544	0	0

Sources: Mangles, R.A., Holden, J.M., Beecher, G.R., Forman, M.R., Lanza, E., "Carotenoid Content of Fruits and Vegetables: An Evaluation of Analytic Data," Journal of the American Dietetic Association 93:3, 284–296, 1993; Marcozzi, M.S., Beecher, G.R., Taylor, P.R., and Khachik, F., Journal of the National Cancer Institute 82, 282–285, 1990.

While most studies have focused on beta-carotene, other carotenoids may be just as—if not more—important, according to Dr. Dexter Morris, vice chair of the Department of Emergency Medicine at the University of North Carolina School of Medicine at Chapel Hill. Lycopene, another member of the carotenoid family, may actually be responsible for many of the health benefits currently attributed to beta-carotene. And it may not be carotenoids at all, but another phytochemical (or group of phytochemicals) altogether that is present in vegetables and fruits that also contain carotenoids.

"The studies regarding the protective effects of certain phytochemicals are enormously consistent and numerous," Taylor says. "So we took the leap and went to carotenoids, then to beta-carotene. There's definitely something there that beta-carotene correlates with in terms of disease prevention. But whether it's beta-carotene, or another carotenoid, or a broad class of phytochemical altogether, we don't know. We do know that phytochemicals in foods have beneficial, disease-preventing effects. But we need to decide whether we want to take it in Mother Nature's package, or in the drug companies' packages."

Many other researchers and nutritionists are also dubious about justifying supplementation, when epidemiological studies indicate that a diet rich in fruits and vegetables can prevent disease. "Why spend a lot of time and effort finding a little pill to take?" Morris says. "Supplements are hit or miss, and mostly they miss. There are a lot of questions, and while we're figuring out the answer, the safest bet is to eat a varied, nutritious diet and be cautious about thinking that taking any one supplement will somehow make your health better."

Other problems with pills include the possibility of toxic reactions and issues of bioavailability. Vitamin A, for example, is extremely toxic if consumed in excess and can cause fatigue, lethargy, abdominal discomfort, headaches, insomnia, night sweats, edema, liver damage, and central nervous system disorders. In large enough doses, vitamin A may be fatal.[2]

One recent study has suggested that pregnant women who take high doses—more than 10,000 IU—of vitamin A increase the risk of serious birth defects in their babies, including cleft lip, cleft palate, fluid on the brain, and heart abnormalities. The study of more than 22,000 women was based only on preformed vitamin A, rather than precursors such as beta-carotene. The researchers emphasized that women were not at risk from consuming tomatoes, carrots, or other foods high in carotenoids.[3]

Some evidence also suggests that vitamin E in large doses may interfere with blood clotting, and extremely high doses (more than 1,200 IU per day) may cause headache, fatigue, weakness, and digestive disorders. Extremely high doses of some water-soluble vitamins, especially niacin (vitamin B_3) and vitamin B_6, may have adverse effects: niacin may cause flushing of the skin, nausea, diarrhea, increased blood glucose levels and changes in liver function. Long-term, excessive consumption of vitamin B_6 (more than 500 to 1,000 mg per day, for more than two years) can cause sensory-nerve damage. And then there's the complicated issue of interaction—both positive and negative—between compounds.[4]

In terms of supplementation, one study found that with beta-carotene supplementation, blood alpha-carotene and lycopene concentrations also went up.[5] "We've speculated that some absorption pathway common to carotenoids exists and that with supplementation with one carotenoid, others may be absorbed generically," Taylor says. "The other possibility is that beta-carotene is quenching free radicals and preserving alpha-carotene and lycopene." A third explanation, according to Anthony Almada, may be that beta-carotene supplementation may cause a redistribution of other carotenoids stored in tissues, shifting them into the blood. Interaction between compounds isn't limited to beta-carotene and the carotenoids—for example, vitamin C may help recycle vitamin E in the body, regenerating it after it has quenched a free-radical reaction.[6]

"Our experience *has* been that higher levels of carotenoids in the blood indicated a lower risk of heart disease" Morris says. "But keep in mind that a lot of different substances in fruits and vegetables may be working in conjunction with those carotenoids. That's why isolated supplements aren't as good an insurance policy as a balanced diet. If you give someone a carrot, they'll be getting beta-carotene. But they'll also get a number of substances that we haven't identified yet."

He points out that all epidemiological studies looking at beta-carotene indicate its protective benefits regarding heart disease and that it may well be that researchers could come up with a cocktail of supplements that are beneficial in preventing heart disease and other illnesses. "But for now," he says, "there is no evidence that supplements, at least for the normal person, are overwhelmingly beneficial, and in some cases may be detrimental."

That detrimental effect has to do with the interaction between phytochemical compounds. "In one study, beta-carotene supplementation interfered with vitamin D absorption—and this was using modest doses of beta-carotene," Morris says. "The problem is, no one knows whether you should have *x* amount of vitamin D and *y* amount of beta-carotene, because no one yet fully understands the interactions. And I'm not sure there ever will be a comprehensive study or answer."

Other researchers also caution against the possible adverse effects of taking large quantities of certain supplements. Lenore Kohlmeier, Ph.D., professor of nutrition and epidemiology at University of North Carolina School of Medicine at Chapel Hill, has advised against taking beta-carotene supplements because of evidence that excessive amounts of beta-carotene may reduce the body's ability to absorb lycopene. "There is precious little real research out there," she says. "I feel so strongly that there's some substance or multiple substances in foods, and we're so ignorant at this point that we'd be foolish to go to supplements. We may get lucky and find safe ingredients that are most

- *Alpha-carotene.* Decreased risk of lung cancer; decreased growth of cancer cells; improved immune response.
- *Beta-carotene.* Decreased risk of lung, colon, bladder, and skin cancers; increased immune response.
- *Canthaxanthin.* Decreased risk of skin cancers; inhibited growth of cancer cells; improved immunity.
- *Lutein.* Decreased risk of lung cancer; protection against heart disease; prevention of macular degeneration.
- *Lycopene.* Decreased risk of prostate, colon, and bladder cancers; decreased growth of cancer cells.

effective when isolated and taken in high doses. But until then, if we look at isolating certain compounds, we may be barking up the wrong tree."

And LaChance advises against taking supplements of individual carotenoids. "In nature, we get a mix of carotenoids, and we don't yet know how important it is to get this mix," he says. "If you take a pill you have no choice. You're only getting one—say, beta-carotene—and it may not be the most important one. It's fine to talk about phytochemicals, but it's going to be a long time before this is a *fait accompli.* There are thousands and thousands of chemicals in foods, and with that many compounds, interactions become a huge factor. We've isolated 52 nutrients, and now we're studying and trying to understand the interaction between those nutrients. If we can't do it with fifty-two, how can we do it with 5,000?" It is estimated that there are more than six hundred carotenoids, and only about thirty are precursors of vitamin A—that is, they are transformed in the body into vitamin A. The functional benefits of carotenoids are likely unrelated to vitamin A but rather to their antioxidant properties.

Low concentrations of beta-carotene in the blood and in the diet are consistently predictive of total mortality, lung cancer, other cancers, and heart disease, according to Taylor. "But when we give people beta-carotene supplements, we see an increase in lung cancer," he says. "Why? There are several possible explanations. We seem to have identified an interaction between alcohol and beta-carotene. That is, those increases in lung cancer were limited to people who drank the most."

Other studies have confirmed these results. "In one study, a group of baboons was given beta-carotene supplements and alcohol, and another group was given alcohol alone," according to Anthony Almada. "And the baboons who received beta-carotene and alcohol showed much more severe liver damage than those that received alcohol alone." Why? No one knows. "We don't know about the true safety of beta-carotene in humans," he says. "And there is no clear answer. There are lines of thinking and levels of education, but there's a big ignorance factor."

Pills certainly can't deliver the same broad range of nutrients, trace elements, and possibly unidentified compounds as whole foods. Nor can they provide us with the fiber, fat, protein, and carbohydrates we need for daily existence—or furnish us with the gustatory pleasure we derive from a satisfying meal. Some far-thinking researchers maintain that it may someday be possible to derive all of our nutritional needs from supplements, but imagine settling down at the dinner table with a pile of pills and a tall glass of water, while fondly remembering fragrant, steaming plates of healthy food. Fortunately, such a scenario doesn't seem likely in our lifetimes.

4

LIVE LONGER, LOOK YOUNGER, FEEL BETTER

 No matter what diets we follow or pills we take, we all die. We can't stop, control, or avoid the fact of our mortality. But we do have some influence over *when* we die, and *how*.

Focusing more on the concept of health span, as opposed to life span, health-care researchers are looking for ways to beat the big killers in the American population—cancer, cardiovascular disease, and hypertension. Additionally, more and more nutrition and health research is focusing on increasing immunity and enhancing performance. Again, it's the live longer, look younger, feel better dream, and more and more research seems to indicate that in fact we can expect to extend the number of years we live healthy, fruitful lives, free of age-related diseases.

Most research seems to indicate that, with the help of the foods we eat and the supplements we take, we can expect to dramatically minimize the risk of the most common causes of death: cancer, cardiovascular disease, and diseases related to obesity. Countless studies have shown the benefits of certain foods in reducing the risk of cancer, heart disease, and hypertension. Compounds in celery help prevent high blood pressure by relaxing the muscles that line blood-vessel walls, thereby widening the vessels. Other foods that help lower blood pressure include garlic and onions, olive oil, grapefruit, fenugreek, and fish oil. A number of studies suggest that regular consumption of garlic and onions helps prevent heart disease by inhibiting the clumping of blood platelets and thus decreasing the likelihood of their deposit on blood-vessel walls. Omega-3 fatty acids, found in cold-water fish such as salmon, tuna, cod, and sardines, have also been shown to prevent abnormal clotting.[1] At the time of this writing, the most comprehensive research in human studies focuses on the antioxidant vitamins—A, C, and E—and on beta-carotene.

In 1994, heart disease and cancer accounted for 70 percent of all deaths in the United States, and most experts estimate that at least a third of cancer cases can be attributed to diet and about half of cardiovascular diseases and hypertension are related to diet.[2]

THE CANCER ANSWER

Cancer is the second leading cause of death in the United States. More than 2 million new cases of all types of cancer will be diagnosed in 1995, and about 547,000 people will die of cancer—almost 1,500 people a day. About 20 percent of all deaths in the United States are from cancer. Additionally, there has been a steady increase in the incidence of mortality from cancer since the mid-1930s, and the numbers have continued to rise consistently.[3]

Table 2

INCIDENCE OF CANCER RATE INCREASES AMONG AMERICANS, 1973 TO 1991

OVERALL CANCER RATE INCREASE: 390 CASES PER 100,000

All sites	22*
Prostate	126
Melanoma	94
Non-Hodgkin's lymphoma	73
Testis	43
Kidney and renal pelvis	35
Lung and bronchus	34
Brain and nervous system	25
Breast	24

*Percentage increase for all ages, for the years between 1973 and 1991

Source: Cancer Facts, SEER Cancer Statistics Review 1973-1991, *National Cancer Institute, National Institutes of Health, Bethesda, MD, 1994*

No one has come up with a definitive answer to what *causes* cancer, but researchers understand the basic mechanisms of the disease. The causal elements of cancer include chemicals, radiation, viruses, and internal elements, such as hormones, immune conditions, and inherited mutations. These factors may act together to initiate carcinogenesis. Cancer cells are rapidly dividing cells that proliferate at abnormal rates of growth. It is now understood that normal cells have sets of genes called protooncogenes, which can be activated by cancer-causing agents and can initiate tumor formation. Some of the more common tumor initiators include nitrosamines, found in many processed foods and cigarette smoke, polychlorinated biphenyls (PCBs), asbestos, ultraviolet radiation, saccharin, excess fat, foods cooked at very high temperatures, and certain hormones.

In terms of cancer prevention through nutrition, whole fruits and vegetables seem to offer the best defense. The cancer risk for Americans who eat the recommended amounts (five servings) of fruits and vegetables (especially dark green, leafy vegetables and red, orange, and yellow fruits and vegetables) on a daily basis is 50 to 70 percent lower than for those who consume the least fruits and vegetables. Research consistently indicates that people who consume the highest quantity of fruits and vegetables are about half as likely to develop cancer as those who consume the least. And dietary changes could result in a reduction of deaths from all cancers by more than a third. The most potent defenders seem to be antioxidant vitamins and phytochemicals. Vitamins A, C, and E and beta-carotene act as antioxidants, destroying harmful free radicals in the body. Vitamins C and E may inhibit the formation of cancer-causing substances in the intestinal tract, and vitamins A, C, and E, and beta-carotene may reduce the action of tumor-promoting agents in the body, stimulate the immune system, and convert cancer cells back to normal cells.[4]

Regarding the role of antioxidants in preventing cancer, Dr. Gladys Block of the University of California at Berkeley has reviewed 130 epidemiological studies and says that "with possibly fewer than five exceptions, every single study is in the protective direction, and something like 110 to 120 studies found statistically significant reduced risk with high intake (of antioxidants)." The antioxidant carotenoids have been linked in numerous studies with decreased risk of lung cancer and cancers of the colon, bladder, prostate, and skin, and decreased growth of cancer cells in mice. These protective nutrients are found in red, orange, and yellow fruits and vegetables such as carrots, tomatoes, and strawberries, and they are converted in the body into vitamin A. In the mid-1960s, a number of preliminary studies began to suggest that vitamin A offers protection against lung cancer. Further research has validated those earlier findings and has focused on members of the carotenoid family, which can act as precursors to vitamin A.

One study of more than 25,000 Japanese men and women indicated a protective effect of beta-carotene against cancers of the lung, stomach,

What we know in 1995 is that diet may play a role in 35 percent of cancer deaths. What we don't know for sure is which constituents either cause or prevent cancer.

Charles Hennekens, professor of medicine at Harvard University, Boston, quoted in the *Wall Street Journal*, May 8, 1995

colon, prostate, and cervix. Dozens of other epidemiological studies since 1985 have consistently pointed to a link between high consumption of dietary beta-carotene and decreased risk of cancer, especially lung cancer. The so-called Western Electric study followed almost 2,000 men for 19 years and compared their incidence of cancer, based on dietary vitamin A and carotenoid intake. Men with the lowest consumption of dietary carotenoids had seven times the incidence of lung cancer compared to those with the highest consumption.[5]

One compelling area of research focuses on the role of beta-carotene and cervical cancer. Studies have found that women with the lowest dietary beta-carotene intake were two to three times more likely to develop cervical cancer or abnormalities in the cervix than those women who consumed the highest amounts of beta-carotene. Women with cervical lesions had lower blood beta-carotene than healthy women in another study, and women with the highest blood beta-carotene had an 80 percent reduction in the risk of cervical cancer. A number of other studies have supported these findings.[6]

Vitamin E, the second member in the trilogy of protective antioxidant vitamins, has also shown promise as a preventive agent against cancer, especially in the way it enables the body to neutralize airborne oxidants such as ozone or cigarette smoke. Vitamin E food sources include nuts, nut and seed oils, wheat germ, and whole wheat. A 1988 study of more than 20,000 men in Finland found that men with the highest blood vitamin E had the lowest risk of cancer—about 70 percent less than those with the lowest vitamin E and only 60 percent the risk of cancers related to smoking.[7]

Again, vitamin E seems to work best in concert with other antioxidants. Vitamin E helps reduce the risk of stomach cancer—especially in conjunction with vitamin C—through its ability to block the formation of nitrosamines, carcinogenic compounds created in the digestive tract. Nitrites and nitrates, found in processed, pickled, cured, and smoked foods, can be turned into nitrosamines in the body, but vitamins E and C can inhibit this conversion. Vitamin E may also enhance the ability of selenium, a trace mineral, to inhibit the development of tumors in the breast.[8]

Vitamin C—found in broccoli, brussels sprouts, oranges, green peppers, and numerous other fruits and vegetables—has also been linked, directly and indirectly, to the prevention of cancer and inhibition of tumor growth. In the mid-1970s, Dr. Linus Pauling, the two-time Nobel laureate and legendary proponent and researcher of vitamin C, studied 1,000 terminally ill cancer patients and found that those who received a daily supplement of 10 grams of vitamin C lived about 4 times longer than 1,000 patients who received no supplements and that some of those who received supplements lived 20 times longer.[9] Pauling later stated that "evidence continues to accumulate that vitamin C has numerous biological effects, including some that may relate to the prevention of cancer."

The *Surgeon General's Report on Nutrition and Health* issued in 1988 concluded that numerous studies did show the protective effect of foods containing vitamin C against cancers of the esophagus, stomach, and cervix.[10] A 1989 report from the National Research Council offered a similar conclusion, citing numerous studies that suggest consumption of fruits and vegetables containing vitamin C may offer protection against cancer.[11]

A number of functional foods and phytochemicals have shown promise in protecting against cancer. Garlic extract has been shown to reduce mammary tumors in animals and to reduce the growth of cultured human melanoma cells, and various garlic preparations have been shown to suppress the formation of nitrosamines in the stomach, inhibit other carcinogens, and reduce the growth of human breast cancer cells. A broad range of human studies show more and more evidence that increased consumption of garlic is related to lower incidence of cancer.[12]

Other compounds that have been shown to help prevent cancer include the following:

- Phytic acid and protease inhibitors in *soybeans* are potential anticarcinogenic compounds
- Lignins, found in *flaxseed oil and other oils, seeds, and grains,* including soybeans, triticale, and wheat, have been shown to inhibit the growth of human breast-cancer cells
- Isothiocyanate compounds in *cruciferous vegetables* may help protect against nitrosamine-induced lung tumors
- Phenolic compounds, including catechins, in *green tea* are related to inhibition of tumor formation in animals
- Other phenolic compounds found in *turmeric* inhibit carcinogenesis and tumor promotion
- Glycyrrhizin, responsible for the sweet flavor in real *licorice root,* may help prevent tumor formation
- Insoluble dietary fiber, found in *whole grains and vegetables,* and *psyllium,* a soluble dietary fiber, appear to inhibit tumor formation

TAKING HEART: CARDIOVASCULAR DISEASE

Cardiovascular disease is the leading cause of death in the United States, accounting for almost 1 million deaths every year—close to twice as many as cancer. According to the American Heart Association, almost one out of every two Americans dies of cardiovascular disease; heart disease kills someone in the United States every 34 seconds. Of the U.S. population of about 255 million people in 1995, almost 59 million had some form of heart disease.

The heart is a non-stop muscle and, like all other muscles in the body, requires a constant exchange of oxygen and nutrients and removal of waste products. Coronary arteries carry oxygen- and nutrient-laden blood to the heart. If the flow of blood is blocked by platelet buildup on the walls of the arteries (atherosclerosis), the arteries thicken and the passageway for blood narrows, reducing the flow of oxygen and nutrients to the heart. Free-radical damage has been found in numerous studies to be related to the development and progression of atherosclerosis, and antioxidants may help prevent heart disease by preventing free-radical damage.

Vitamin E, found in nuts, nut and seed oils, wheat germ, and whole wheat, seems to be the most efficacious of the antioxidants in preventing heart disease. At high dosages (400 or more IU per day), vitamin E apparently helps prevent atherosclerosis, perhaps by inhibiting oxidation of LDL (the bad cholesterol) levels. One eight-year study of more than 87,000 American women showed that the risk of heart disease was 36.5 percent lower in those women who had begun taking more than 100 IU per day of vitamin E in supplement form, compared to women who did not take vitamin E. For women who took vitamin E for more than two years, the risk was about 50 percent less.[13] The reason for vitamin E's efficacy in reducing the risk of heart disease may be in its tendency to prevent atherosclerosis. Studies have consistently shown that vitamin E can reduce the likelihood of developing atherosclerosis, by inhibiting the tendency of blood platelets to clump together and by stimulating the production of prostacyclin, a hormone-like product from fatty acids, which inhibits platelet aggregation.[14]

Beta-carotene also shows great promise in protecting against heart disease: in one study, women with high consumption of beta-carotene had a 22 percent lower risk of heart disease. In another study, men who took beta-carotene supplements were half as likely to die of heart disease.[15]

Dexter Morris, of the University of North Carolina School of Medicine at Chapel Hill, examined the concentrations of various carotenoids in the blood of almost 2,000 middle-aged men with high blood cholesterol and a high risk of heart disease and over a 13-year period found that those with the highest blood carotenoids were a third less likely to have heart attacks. "We looked at the whole group of men and compared those with the highest levels of serum carotenoids with those who had the lowest levels," Morris says. "Those in the highest categories had 35 percent fewer heart attacks or deaths from heart attacks than those in the lowest categories." In a similar study, Morris's University of North Carolina colleague Lenore Kohlmeier found that men who had suffered heart attacks generally had lower beta-carotene concentrations in their body fat than men who had not suffered heart attacks.

Vitamin C, found in green peppers, broccoli, tomatoes, citrus, and a variety of other fruits and vegetables, has shown some promise in the prevention of heart disease. One study found that men with the highest vitamin C intake were almost half as likely to die from heart disease than those with lower vitamin C intake (less than 50 mg per day). Other research has shown that vitamin C can decrease LDL-cholesterol levels and increase HDL-cholesterol levels, an important factor in heart disease.[16]

A number of phytochemical compounds have been shown to help prevent certain types of heart disease. More than 400 foods and herbs are known to have anti-occlusive (preventing the narrowing or blockage of blood vessels) and anti-atherosclerotic effects on the heart. Thioallyl compounds found in garlic have been shown to have a vast range of heart-protective effects, including lowering blood cholesterol, reducing blood clotting, and inhibiting platelet aggregation and adhesion. *Ginkgo biloba*—the gingko tree, whose leaves, seeds, and nuts have been used in traditional medicine for years—has been shown to stimulate blood circulation, significantly improve the condition of coronary-heart-disease patients, and lower blood cholesterol.[17]

Catechins in green tea may help strengthen capillary walls and protect against heart disease, and omega-3 fatty acids in cold-water fish such as salmon and cod have long been known to have a protective effect against cardiovascular disease by preventing atherosclerosis. Some members of the flavonoid family have been used to treat atherosclerosis and myocardial infarction.[18] A number of other "novel" compounds are also thought to help protect against heart disease, including:

- astragalus
- bilberry
- ginseng
- chromium
- co-Q 10
- medicinal mushrooms

FIGHTING FAT: OBESITY AND HYPERTENSION

For years, Americans have been waging a seemingly fruitless war against growing waistlines and increasingly higher digits on their bathroom scales.

In a 13-year study with 1,899 men, we found that, among people who had never smoked, those with the highest blood levels of beta-carotene had 70 percent fewer heart attacks or deaths from heart attacks than those in the lowest quartile.

Dr. Dexter Morris, vice chair of the Department of Emergency Medicine at the University of North Carolina School of Medicine, Chapel Hill

Sadly enough, most of the focus and fervor has been on the cosmetic benefits, rather than the health benefits, of being thin. As researchers continue to amass information about the deleterious effects of obesity, they are finding that the old adage "You can never be too rich or too thin" may at least be half true.

Obesity is defined by the American Heart Association (AHA) as an excessive accumulation of body fat, and a person is considered obese when body weight exceeds the so-called desirable weight for height and gender by 20 percent or more and when that excess weight is fat, rather than water, muscle, or bone. Desirable weight is based on the outdated 1959 Metropolitan Life weight tables, but the AHA continues to use these as a format although the insurance industry revised ideal weight upward by almost 10 percent in 1983.

The dangers of obesity are many, and costly, totaling about $68.8 billion per year in the United States. Obesity is a factor in 19 percent of all cases of heart disease, 30 percent of gallbladder diseases, and 2.3 percent of cancers. It raises blood cholesterol and blood pressure, lowers HDL (the good cholesterol) levels, and can induce diabetes. Additionally, obesity costs the nation $23 billion in a number of indirect costs, including lost productivity and wages as a result of hospitalization and early death.[19]

Researchers have spent considerable time focusing on caloric intake and caloric restriction, examining their effects on overall health and disease prevention, and the results have been compelling. Several epidemiological studies have shown a correlation between caloric intake and increased risk of cancer, and caloric restriction has been shown to help inhibit or delay the formation and development of tumors. Cancers and tumors of the skin, breast, lung, liver, colon, pancreas, muscle, lymphatic system, and endocrine system may be deterred by caloric restriction.[20]

Other points to note include that the longer you're fat, the more danger you're in. A lifetime of obesity exerts continuous stress on the heart, causing physical changes in the size and shape of the heart and increasing the risk of heart attack. Additionally, the distribution of fat seems to play a role in the danger of obesity: physicians and nutritionists warn that a heavy distribution of fat in the belly, rather than the hips, thighs, or other parts of the body, has repeatedly been linked to increased risk of heart disease.

Obesity and extreme overweight tend to raise cholesterol and triglycerides—the major type of fat that circulates in the blood—and contribute to hypertension. Hypertension, or high blood pressure, is the most dangerous direct consequence of obesity, affecting nearly 50 million Americans in 1995. Hypertension alone was responsible for more than 35,000 deaths in 1992 and contributed to thousands more deaths through stroke, heart attack, and heart failure, according to the American Heart Association. The causes and effects of hypertension are tied together in a complicated web. Hypertension is related to obesity, which is related to excessive caloric and fat intake, which is related to elevated cholesterol levels, which are related to the formation of atherosclerosis walls, which increases the likelihood of hypertension.

And while the exact cause of 90 to 95 percent of high blood pressure isn't known, those agents that tend to aggravate or create a predisposition to high blood pressure have been recognized for years. Factors contributing to hypertension include obesity, excessive fat intake, stress, genetic predisposition, sodium sensitivity, imbalanced magnesium and potassium levels, lack of exercise, and cigarette smoking. Pack-a-day cigarette smokers, for example, are twice as likely to have hypertension and heart attacks as nonsmokers.[21]

Hypertension is a major factor in heart disease, weakening arterial and venous vessel walls, leading to aneurysms that can lead to heart attack, and contributing to congestive heart failure.[22] A number of studies suggest that hypertension is related to free radicals and those diseases caused by free radicals. Some researchers postulate that free radicals block the production of substances that help relax blood vessels and therefore reduce blood pressure. High blood levels of vitamin C and selenium have been related to lower blood pressure, and vitamin C alone has been shown to help in reducing high blood pressure.[23]

LIVING STRONGER, LIVING LONGER

Immunity

While we Americans are deluged on a daily basis with facts about cancer, heart disease, hypertension, and other fatal conditions, the fact is that most of us are at least as concerned in the short run with the latter portion of the "live longer, look younger, feel better" equation. We may watch our diets, exercise regularly, and monitor our stress and cholesterol levels with the intention of preventing fatal disease. But on a day-to-day basis we're just as, if not more, interested in preventing common colds, hay fever, bladder infections, and all the many other irritating allergies, viruses, and bacterial infections that can plague our everyday lives. Hence the focus of research and media attention. We may all want to live to be 100, but we also want to be stronger and more physically invincible right now.

Our bodies are equipped with a vast array of defense mechanisms, designed to provide us with some immunity to deleterious external factors, including bacteria, viruses, environmental pollutants, and so forth. This immune system serves us in two ways: it disables harmful external factors, and it repairs damaged tissue and cells. Sometimes, however, our systems are over-

In 1990, more than 400,000 Americans died of smoking-related illnesses. Almost 20 percent of deaths from heart disease are attributable to smoking. It's also estimated that almost 40,000 nonsmokers died from heart diseases as a result of exposure to environmental tobacco smoke.

American Heart Association, *Heart and Stroke Facts: 1995 Statistical Supplement.*

loaded by external factors—a poor diet, cigarette smoking, or exposure to toxic chemicals—and the circuits blow. Our immune system is unable to keep up or it gets revved up too high—and we get sick.

Much research has been done on the role of antioxidants and phytochemicals in enhancing the immune system, and the results are fairly consistent: antioxidant vitamins and certain phytochemicals can dramatically boost the immune system, reducing the body's vulnerability to external influences and internal malfunctioning. Antioxidants have been shown in numerous studies to dramatically enhance immune-system function.

Vitamin A can lower the rate of infections, and high doses of beta-carotene can increase T-cell (T-lymphocytes, a type of white blood cell involved in immune function) numbers. A deficiency of vitamin A has been shown in numerous studies to significantly increase the risk of infection, especially in children, and vitamin A has also been shown to have a protective effect against environmental pollutants, including second-hand smoke, carbon monoxide, and ozone.[24] Beta-carotene, which is converted in the body into vitamin A, has been shown to enhance overall immune response. In terms of dosage, 180 mg per day of beta-carotene has been shown to increase the rate at which the body produces protective T-cells.[25]

Vitamin E enhances various facets of the immune system, most likely by protecting vulnerable white blood cells from oxidative damage. In combination with selenium, vitamin E contributes to increased immune-system function, especially when it is taken in amounts of about 400 IU per day in supplement form. Additionally, vitamin E can retard age-related immune decline.[26]

Perhaps the most celebrated vitamin in terms of immune enhancement is vitamin C. Because vitamin C is water soluble, it's able to attack free radicals in the watery portions in and between cells, before they're able to affect the cell membrane and other fat-based portions of the cells. Studies have confirmed the efficacy of vitamin C in immune enhancement, showing that it can stimulate the production of white blood cells, help the liver detoxify chemicals, and inactivate a variety of viruses and bacteria.

Celebrated as a miracle drug for fighting the common cold by its earliest proponent, Linus Pauling, vitamin C may be the most easily available and potent immune enhancer. Studies have found that administration of large doses of vitamin C is related to increased immune function.[27] At the same time, deficiency in vitamin C is associated with decreased antibacterial function of macrophages—scavenger cells that remove bacteria and other foreign bodies from blood and cells—and with decreased resistance to infection.[28] Additionally, vitamin C can promote faster healing: post-operative patients

IMMUNITY ENHANCERS

Manganese Found in pineapple, oatmeal, whole grains, nuts and seeds, beans, spinach, tea, vegetables

Zinc Found in herring, wheat germ, sesame seeds, blackstrap molasses, soybeans, sunflower seeds, beets, walnuts, beans, avocados, millet, brown rice, almonds

Co-Q10 Found in sardines, mackerel, peanuts, pistachios, soybeans, walnuts, sesame seeds

Selenium Found in Brazil nuts, tuna, swordfish, seafood, whole grains, sunflower seeds, liver, broccoli, mushrooms, cabbage, celery

Flavonoids Found in broccoli, cauliflower, cabbage, brussels sprouts, citrus fruits, nuts, seeds, beans, onions, garlic

Ginseng A Chinese herb used in the Orient for cooking and medicinal purposes, and said to be energizing; contains a number of healthy compounds, including saponin, ginsenin, panoxic, panaxin, and panaquilon

Astragalus A Chinese herb used in the Orient for cooking and medicinal purposes, and said to be strengthening and warming

Lentinan Found exclusively in shiitake mushrooms

Beta-carotene Found in carrots, mangos, cantaloupes, persimmons, apricots, watermelon, red pepper, pumpkin, greens, spinach, broccoli, winter squash, sweet potatoes, yams, parsley, endive, pimentos, nectarines, papayas

Thiols Found primarily in garlic, onions, radishes, horseradish, mustards

Vitamin A Found in cod-liver oil, liver, swordfish, whitefish, and other fish

Vitamin C Found in acerola cherries, guavas, black currants, parsley, green peppers, watercress, chives, strawberries, persimmons, spinach, oranges, cabbage, grapefruit, papayas, elderberries, kumquats, dandelion greens, cantaloupes, lemons, green onions, limes, mangos, loganberries, tangerines, tomatoes, squash, raspberries, pineapples

Vitamin E Found in wheat germ, safflower oil, nuts, seeds, whole wheat, sesame oil, olive oil, cabbage, cod-liver oil, soy lecithin, spinach, asparagus, broccoli, parsley, oats, barley, corn

---

or those with injuries have been shown to recover 50 to 70 times faster with a daily intake of 400 to 3,000 mg of vitamin C.[29]

Some of the best food sources for boosting immunity include shiitake mushrooms and garlic.[30] Shiitake mushrooms are a wonderful departure from traditional button mushrooms—try the Smoky Shiitake-Brussels Sprouts Salad or the Basil-Lentil Stew in the recipe section. And garlic has long been recognized as having antiviral and antibacterial properties. The active substances in garlic can stimulate the activity of T-cells and macrophages, and garlic is easy and delicious in almost any recipe—try the Lentil-Garlic Paté or Garlic Hummus with Roasted Red Peppers.

Enhanced performance and stamina

Perhaps one more aspiration should be added to the live longer, look younger, feel better model: work harder. Or, in the succinct words of the Nike company, immortalized on T-shirts across the United States, "Eat right. Get lots of sleep. Drink plenty of fluids. Go like hell." In our get-up-and-go, just-do-it culture, we want to climb mountains and bike across countries and feel fantastic in the process. Hundreds of thousands of Americans, in their quests for bigger biceps, flatter tummies, and faster running speeds, have turned to nutrition for assistance in pursuing the elusive goal of physical perfection, of reaching peak performance with enhanced stamina and increased endurance. We *can* climb mountains and win marathons and bike from coast to coast. But not without the right diet and optimum nutrition.

A number of compounds are believed to enhance that elusive mega-endurance goal: octacosanol, found primarily in wheat germ; spirulina, a type of blue-green algae; bee pollen; Siberian ginseng; L-carnitine; and creatine are all thought to enhance overall physical stamina, energy, and endurance. While relatively little hard data exist to support claims of enhanced physical performance as a direct result of diet or supplements, some compelling research exists for a number of compounds, including antioxidant vitamins, that may be of special benefit to athletes.

No story worth telling is complete without a bit of controversy. In this case, it's between two camps that disagree on the effect of increased free radicals during vigorous, intense exercise. Exhaustive exercise is believed by some researchers to increase the production of free radicals by the mitochondria. Oxygen uptake is higher during vigorous exercise, and free-radical levels in muscle and liver tissue may increase dramatically. And wherever more oxygen exists, more free radicals are also present, thus increasing the likelihood of damage to cells.[31]

The good news is that vitamin E may help protect the body from possible oxidative damage caused by excessive exercise. "The implication is that any long-term deleterious effects that may be caused by extreme exercise can be minimized by antioxidants," says Lester Packer, a professor in the Department of Molecular and Cell Biology at the University of California at Berkeley. "In the long run, that may be important to health, and important to overall performance. The cumulative damage that would be associated with exercise may be minimized by vitamin E."

Some experts argue the theory that exercise induces harmful free-radical production in the first place: "In terms of claims that excessive exercise causes muscle damage, you're talking about a big leap of faith," replies Anthony Almada, who contends that there is nothing to suggest that among a group of physically active individuals, exercise is harmful. On the contrary, says Almada, the totality of the evidence points to the fact that regular and vigorous exercise over the lifetime has a protective effect on the body.

The answer to these seemingly conflicting points of view may lie in the body's ability to adapt to stress. The apparently deleterious effects of exhaustive exercise may have to do with the "weekend warrior" syndrome—that is, people who are not on a regular exercise program but who exercise vigorously and sporadically may be more prone to oxidative stress factors. Conversely, regular exercise produces adaptive antioxidant effects in the body and makes the body more able to tolerate muscle stress. With regular exer-

BRAIN FOOD

Ginkgo An extract made from the leaves of the *Ginkgo biloba* tree; helps relieve memory loss and depression

Boron A trace mineral that may positively affect the brain's electrical activity; found in nuts, fruits, legumes, and leafy vegetables

Thiamin Vitamin B_1, known as the nerve vitamin; low levels have been linked to impaired brain activity; found in wheat germ, wheat bran, and nuts

Riboflavin Vitamin B_2; helps improve memory; found in liver, milk, and almonds

Iron High levels appear to boost brain-wave activity; found in greens, liver, shellfish, red meat, and soy products

Zinc Marginal deficiencies can impair mental function and memory; found in seafood, legumes, and whole grains.

Co-Q 10 An essential coenzyme for metabolism; may help prevent degenerative brain disease, such as Alzheimer's, as well as age-related loss of memory and brain function; found in sardines, mackerel, peanuts, pistachios, soybeans, walnuts, and sesame seeds

Folic acid A B vitamin responsible for the formation of red blood cells; believed to prevent deterioration of mental function, including memory loss and dementia; found in leafy greens, beans, seeds, and liver.

Sources: Jean Carper, Food: Your Miracle Medicine, *New York: HarperCollins Publishers, 1993; Jean Carper,* Stop Aging Now!, *New York: HarperCollins Publishers, 1995; and Harold M. Silverman, Joseph A. Romano, and Gary Elmer,* The Vitamin Book, *New York: Bantam, 1985*

cise, tolerance levels increase, pain thresholds increase, and muscle strength increases. In other words, what doesn't kill you makes you strong.

In the area of enhanced mental acuity and clarity, the body of data is less concrete but immensely compelling. Brain-power foods and supplements are believed to have a positive effect on everything from warding off Alzheimer's disease, to helping students pass history exams. Some studies have shown that vitamin E can slow progression of nervous-system disorders, possibly offering protection against Alzheimer's and Parkinson's disease. Carotenoids may also have a positive effect on mental alertness: even slight deficiencies of carotenoids and other vitamins can slow mental functioning, while adequate amounts of carotenoids can enhance cognitive function.[32]

The Fanfare about Free Radicals

Given the voluminous amount of research involving antioxidant vitamins and their major role in boosting imune response and reducing the risk of disease, it's worth taking a moment to talk a bit more about free radicals and the role of antioxidants in health.

Free radicals are unstable chemicals formed in the body during normal metabolic processes and from exposure to external sources of toxins such as cigarette smoke and air pollution; antioxidants quench free radicals before they can attack healthy cells and contribute to degenerative diseases: that's the quick version. The longer tale encompasses a complex web of metabolic activities and addresses why free radicals are at the root of many or most diseases and are a major factor in aging.

Table 3

MAJOR ANTIOXIDANT VITAMINS

VITAMIN A: RETINOL

In ancient Egypt, symptoms of night blindness were treated by placing fried liver—rich in vitamin A—over the eyes, and Hippocrates later recommended eating liver as a cure for night blindness. Vitamin A is found in two forms: retinol and carotene. Retinol, from meat sources, can be absorbed as it is by the body. Carotenoids must be broken down by the body before they can be used as vitamin A. The name "fat-soluble A" was originally given to a compound found in egg yolk and butterfat that was determined to be essential for normal growth. Researchers later recognized that yellow pigments (carotenes) in plant substances were also converted in the body into vitamin A.

- *What it does:* essential for good night vision, healthy skin, production of RNA, normal bone growth, cellular integrity, and skeletal and tooth development.
- *Best food sources:* organ meats, egg yolks, butter, fish-liver oil, swordfish, and whitefish.
- *Recommended dose:* 800 to 20,000 IU per day.

VITAMIN C: ASCORBIC ACID

The effects of vitamin C deficiency were first noted among sailors, whose long voyages at sea meant that they were deprived for months of fresh fruits and vegetables. They developed curious and devastating symptoms that included swollen, bleeding gums and the inability of wounds to heal—disease symptoms that were later named scurvy.

- *What it does:* boosts immune function, promotes collagen formation and development, protects against blood clotting and bruising, promotes the healing of wounds, maintains blood-vessel integrity and adrenal-gland function, aids in the production of various hormones and enzymes.
- *Best food sources:* oranges, tangerines, tomatoes, squash, mangos, cantaloupes, spinach, persimmons, brussels sprouts, guavas, strawberries, green peppers, black currants, parsley, watercress, cabbage, grapefruit.
- *Recommended dose:* 60 to 15,000 mg per day.

VITAMIN E: TOCOPHEROL

Researchers in the 1920s found that vitamin E was essential to the ability of pregnant animals to carry to term and necessary for reproduction in general. The other name for vitamin E, tocopherol, thus comes from the Greek words *tokos,* meaning "birth," and *pheros* meaning "to carry."

Table 3, continued

Vitamin E: Tocopherol

- *What it does:* improves circulation, helps repair damaged tissues, promotes normal blood clotting and healing, reduces scarring, helps prevent cataracts and may prevent age spots.
- *Best food sources:* wheat germ, whole grains, sesame, safflower, corn, soy, and peanut oil, nuts and seeds, cabbage, spinach, asparagus, broccoli.
- *Recommended dose:* 30 to 400 IU per day.

Bits and pieces of assorted theories and ideas regarding the role of antioxidants and free radicals in disease are rampant. If you've even briefly perused the health and lifestyle sections of any major newspaper, you've encountered some bit of information about antioxidants over your morning toast and tea or coffee and bagel.

Even though they're a part of the body's natural chemistry, oxidants can injure vital cell structures, destroying DNA, enzymes, proteins, and membranes if they exist at higher levels than normal—a condition usually brought about by environmental pollution, low levels of antioxidants, or inflammatory disease states such as arthritis. At the same time, free radicals are essential for our survival. Our immune systems produce free radicals and pro-oxidants to destroy harmful microorganisms, and free radicals are crucial in producing hormones and activating certain enzymes. Thus, the double-edged sword of free radicals: you can't live with them, and you can't live without them.

In the simplest of terms, free radicals are unstable molecules with unpaired electrons. Chemical compounds are made up of two or more elements held together by a chemical bond. In the body, molecules are held together by electrons. But if a molecule has an unpaired electron, it becomes highly unstable and reactive. This unstable molecule, or "free radical," will then pair with an electron from a stable molecule, thus creating another free radical and starting a dangerous chain that continues indefinitely, unless something intervenes—and that's where antioxidants come in.

Our bodies have natural, built-in control systems to protect against free-radical damage, by removing free radicals with the use of enzymes, scavengers, and antioxidants. Enzymes inactivate free radicals by using them to generate safer chemical reactions. Nonenzymatic scavengers deactivate and trap free radicals, stopping the deleterious chain reaction. And antioxidants control and minimize free-radical reactions in the body's cells.

BREATHE DEEP— CAREFULLY

A seeming paradox in the tale of free radicals involves the role of oxygen. Yes, oxygen is vital to every living cell in the body—but it can also be the cause of degenerative disease. We've all seen the effects of oxidative damage, in everything from rusted cars to rancid butter. And the same thing can happen in our bodies. We've been brought up to believe in oxygen as a life-giving force. But in the body, oxygen can enter into an unstable form, yielding a variety of highly reactive molecules referred to as pro-oxidants, including the following:

- *Superoxide.* A free radical that consists of one oxygen molecule and one electron.
- *Hydroxyl radical.* Made up of equal parts of hydrogen and oxygen, this is the most destructive type of free radical.
- *Hydrogen peroxide.* Able to pass through cell membranes and destroy the interior of cells; although not a free radical itself, this molecule can react with superoxide to form a hydroxyl radical.
- *Lipid peroxy radical.* A free radical formed when oxygen reacts with fatty acids in cell membranes, causing them to release more free radicals and setting off a devastating chain reaction.
- *Singlet oxygen.* Another non-free radical pro-oxidant, composed of an oxygen molecule with two "hyperactive" electrons existing in an unstable conformation in the molecule.

Antioxidants work by patrolling different territories in the body. Enzymes and vitamins protect the cells' internal structures, and antioxidant nutrients can also circulate through the blood to neutralize free radicals outside the cells. Antioxidant enzymes are for the most part genetically predetermined, but dietary deficiencies of certain minerals needed to synthesize enzymes—such as zinc, copper, manganese, and selenium—can inhibit the formation of enzymes. The concentrations of antioxidant nutrients in the body are determined by dietary consumption.

We have looked at the capacity of antioxidant vitamins A, C, and E, beta-carotene, and other substances, to help prevent disease and enhance immunity and performance. Other vitamins that may be beneficial in inhibiting free-radical proliferation include the following:

- *Biotin.* Also known as vitamin H, biotin is a sulfur-containing compound that's important in the metabolism of carbohydrates and fat. Biotin is found in legumes, nuts, egg yolks, brewer's yeast, soybeans, cereals, and grains. The daily requirement is 100 to 200 mcg.
- *Folic acid.* Also called folacin, this compound works closely with vitamin B_{12} and is essential in the production of red blood cells. Folic acid is found primarily in legumes, whole grains, and leafy green vegetables. The daily requirement is 50 to 400 mcg.
- *Pantothenic acid.* Also called vitamin B_5, pantothenic acid is a water-soluble vitamin that has a central role in cellular metabolism. Pantothenic acid is found in rice and other grains, nuts, and legumes. The daily requirement is 4 to 7 mg.

5

THE DYNAMIC DOZEN

The Twelve Best Places to Find Your Phytos

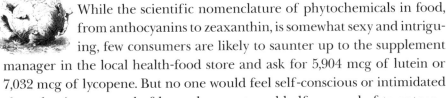 While the scientific nomenclature of phytochemicals in food, from anthocyanins to zeaxanthin, is somewhat sexy and intriguing, few consumers are likely to saunter up to the supplement manager in the local health-food store and ask for 5,904 mcg of lutein or 7,032 mcg of lycopene. But no one would feel self-conscious or intimidated about buying a pound of brussels sprouts and half a pound of tomatoes—which amounts to the same thing, in terms of phytochemical content. Therein lies the sum and substance of the phytochemical advantage: it's not necessary to venture far into the forests of arcane scientific nomenclature. We can discuss the healing benefits of the best-researched phytochemicals in terms of the foods that contain them—since our concern is, after all, meals that heal.

To briefly review definitions and applications, phytochemicals are substances that occur naturally in plants and have the ability to prevent or cure disease. *Thiolallyl compounds* in garlic, for example, have been shown to retard tumor growth and inhibit blood clotting, while *flavonoids and indoles* in a wide variety of cruciferous vegetables have been shown to inhibit cholesterol production and help prevent cancer. Unfortunately, at the time of this writing few significant human studies have been conducted on individual phytochemicals because researchers aren't in agreement about what each of those compounds does, should do, or even is. "Phytochemicals are hardly even discovered," says Rutgers professor Paul LaChance. "In terms of names, we have nothing but bits and pieces—there's no comprehensive picture. There are thousands and thousands of chemicals in food. . . . And while it may be

Tomatoes: vitamin C, vitamin A, glutathione, *p*-coumaric acid, chlorogenic acid, carotenoids (including lycopene)

Cruciferous veggies: vitamin C, vitamin A, sulforaphane, indoles (including indole-3-carbinol), folic acid, fiber, isothiocyanates

Soybeans: isoflavones, genistein, phytic acid, protease inhibitors, phytoestrogens

Whole grains: phenolic acid, phytic acid, vitamin E, fiber (including lignins)

Citrus fruits: vitamin C, terpenes (including limonoids), glutathione

Greens: vitamin C, vitamin A, folic acid, carotenoids (including lutein and beta-carotene)

Red/orange/yellow fruits: vitamin C, vitamin A, fiber, phenols, (including ellagic acid), carotenoids (including beta-carotene, alpha-carotene, lutein, cryptoxanthin, lycopene, zeaxanthin, canthaxanthin)

Red/orange/yellow veggies: vitamin C, vitamin A, fiber, phenols (including ellagic acid), carotenoids (including beta-carotene, alpha-carotene, lutein, cryptoxanthin, lycopene, zeaxanthin, canthaxanthin)

Fish: omega-3 fatty acid, vitamin A

Nuts and seeds: lignins, phenols (including ellagic acid), isoflavones, vitamin E, fatty acids

Beans and legumes: isoflavonoids, phytate, fiber (including lignins), folic acid

Onions and garlic: organosulfur compounds (including allylic sulfides), flavonoids (including quercetin), coumarin, ellagic acid

fine to talk about these substances in general terms, nutritionists still disagree on many of the finer points. In the interim, we're looking at a sort of rank order. We say certain foods seem to be better than others, then make educated guesses."

So while scientists may face an exquisitely complex puzzle in defining which phytos function for what, they recognize that these elusive substances—available in fruits, vegetables, oils, fish and whole grains—can be remarkably potent in the promotion of health and prevention of disease.

The best way to examine and understand phytochemicals and their role in health promotion and disease prevention is by understanding them in terms of the food we put on our plates. Hence the following "dynamic dozen" foods: the phytochemicals and other nutrients they contain will add a spring to your step, a sparkle to your eyes, and possibly quality years to your life.

TOMATOES

The beleaguered tomato, once thought to be a poisonous fruit, has seen its share of bad press. One of its original names was *mala insana*, meaning "unhealthy fruit." Herbalists in the early 1600s said of tomatoes, "The fruit being eaten, it provoketh loathing and vomiting."

Tomatoes have proven their reputation wrong, and the French were more on target in referring to tomatoes as *pommes d'amours*, or love apples.[1] In modern times, these rich fruits—often mistakenly classified as vegetables—have been shown to offer numerous health benefits, with their high concentrations of vitamin C, lycopene, and other nutritious compounds.

A 1985 study at Harvard University by Graham Colditz, M.D., found that older Americans who ate ample amounts of tomatoes were half as likely to die from all forms of cancer as those who didn't consume tomatoes. And tomatoes may even slow the progression of already-developed cancers. In a study of almost 700 men and women with lung cancer at the Cancer Research Center in Hawaii, researchers found that among men, tomatoes were one of the vegetables that nearly doubled the participants' survival time after being diagnosed with cancer.[2]

Many of the health benefits of tomatoes have been attributed to the phytochemical called lycopene, a member of the carotenoid family. Lycopene is relatively rare in foods, and tomatoes are one of only a few foods rich in this potent antioxidant.

Lycopene is thought to help maintain mental and physical functioning as we age and to reduce the risk of pancreatic and cervical cancer. In one study by Dr. David Snowden at the University of Kentucky, older women with the lowest blood concentrations of lycopene scored the lowest on mental and physical functioning tests. Other compounds in tomatoes—*p*-coumaric acid and chlorogenic acid—help to inhibit the formation of nitrosamines. And tomatoes also contain ample amounts of glutathione, a powerful antioxidant that may ward off cancer, help maintain immune function, and help prevent macular degeneration.

These are all good reasons to add more *pommes d'amours* to your daily diet. Eat fresh, juicy tomatoes drizzled with a little olive oil and chopped basil, pour tomato sauces over whole-grain noodles, and warm up rich soups and stews with a tomato base. Tomatoes are one of the best food insurance policies against degenerative disease.

CRUCIFEROUS VEGETABLES

So you still don't like broccoli and brussels sprouts? Get used to them. These members of the Cruciferae family—which also includes cauliflower, cabbage, broccoflower, kale, bok choy, rutabagas, turnips, collard greens, and mustard greens—are packed with phytochemicals that can prevent various types of cancer. "Cruciferous" vegetables, which include plants of the genus *Brassica*, take their name from their "cross-shaped" flower petals.

Sulforaphane in broccoli stimulates the production of anticancer enzymes, which can block the growth of tumors or keep the number and size of existing tumors in check. A compound similar in chemical structure to sulforaphane, cyanohydroxybutene (CHB), may help prevent pancreatic cancer, one of the most deadly forms of cancer, by enhancing the body's ability to neutralize toxins and speed their excretion. The folic acid in crucifers is believed to help prevent colon cancer and precancerous colon polyps.[3]

Cruciferous vegetables also contain indoles, especially indole-3-carbinol, that may help prevent breast cancer. Indole-3-carbinol is thought to increase the production of enzymes that deactivate toxins in food. H. Leon Bradlow, Ph.D., director of biomedical endocrinology at the Strang Cornell Cancer Research Center in New York, reports that women who consume crucifers four times a week can dramatically decrease the production of certain forms of estrogen that are related to breast cancer and cancer of the ovaries and cervix.[4] In another study, people who ate cabbage at least once a week had only a third the risk for colon cancer as those who ate cabbage once a month. But note that indole compounds in crucifers are easily lost in cooking water, so eat them either lightly steamed or raw.

Cruciferous vegetables also contain ample amounts of fiber, as well as the antioxidant vitamins A and C. In terms of vitamin C content, oranges pale in comparison to broccoli. A mere half cup of broccoli contains two-thirds of the RDA for vitamin C. So get used to broccoli and brussels sprouts. Add side dishes of a variety of steamed crucifers to your meals every day, or toss a handful of raw, chopped broccoli into your salads.

SOYBEANS

If your nose turns up and your tastebuds turn off at the mention of soybeans—perhaps you immediately think of tofu—you might want to remind yourself of two compelling reasons to eat these nutrition-packed beans. First, soy has been shown to lower blood cholesterol levels, decrease the risk of heart disease, prevent certain kinds of cancer, and actually help cancerous cells to revert to normal cells. Second, the soybean is available in dozens of different forms, from tempeh and veggie burgers to soy milks and cheeses, that are the bases for a host of infinitely palatable meals. You're not stuck with plain old tofu—so no more excuses.

Soy protein has been shown to reduce both overall cholesterol levels and LDL (the bad cholesterol) levels, without affecting the levels of HDL (the good cholesterol)—thereby helping to prevent heart disease. In one study of 740 people, the consumption of soy protein led to a drop in total cholesterol levels of 9 percent, LDL levels by 13 percent, and triglycerides by 11 percent. The overall drop was the most pronounced in those people with the highest cholesterol levels to begin with.[5]

A compound in soybeans called genistein—a type of isoflavone—appears not only to prevent cancer, but also to cause cancerous cells to differentiate, or revert to normal cells: genistein has been found to repress the growth of almost every kind of cancer cell, including breast, colon, lung, prostate, skin, and leukemia, and to inhibit the progress of already-formed tumors—meaning that soy products could be useful in treating, as well as preventing, cancer. Numerous epidemiological studies have confirmed that countries with the highest consumption of soy have the lowest rates of cancer—including breast, stomach, colon, rectal, lung, and prostate cancer—adjusting for all other factors.[6]

Another compound in soybeans, phytate, has been found to inhibit colon and breast cancer, and is a potent free-radical blocker. Excess iron generates free-radical production, and phytate has been found to bind excess iron in the intestines. The free-radical inhibiting actions of phytate have also been linked to prevention or amelioration of a variety of other diseases, including breast and colon cancer, diabetes, arthritis, and numerous age-related illnesses. Protease inhibitors—substances that interfere with the digestion of protein—help to prevent numerous forms of cancer, including breast, skin, bladder, colon, lung, pancreas, mouth, and esophagus. And so-called phytoestrogens—compounds in the isoflavone family—in soy products may also help relieve hot flashes in menopausal women.[7]

So many different varieties of soy products exist—from hearty tempeh to mellow miso—that the excuses for avoiding soy aren't valid. The health benefits are just too great to ignore.

Whole Grains

Grains are called the staff of life, and for good reason. About 70 percent of the world's population subsists mainly on grains. Grains come in an amazing array of shapes, sizes, colors, and tastes—from the basic wheat and oats to the more exotic varieties, like quinoa, kamut, and spelt—and they're packed with vitamin E, fiber, and other nutritious compounds. And while we may no longer be plagued by beriberi and pellegra, we are besieged by devastating death rates from diseases like cancer that might be prevented with proper nutrition.

Not all grains are the same. Noshing on pasty white bagels for breakfast won't fulfill your fiber needs. Essential oils, trace minerals, and fiber exist in the bran and germ, and the refining process removes these crucial nutritional elements. Whole grains—meaning unprocessed, intact grains that have not had their bran and germ removed—are the variety that contain a wealth of healthy compounds. Grains have been shown to have a preventive effect against colon cancer, by virtue of their fiber content as well as their high concentrations of phytate. Phytate may halt the early stages of breast cancer, possibly by inhibiting the cancer process by binding excess iron in the intestine, and it appears to have a protective effect against cancer of the large intestine, again by binding excess iron.[8] The foods with the highest phytate concentrations include wheat bran, soy flour, and wheat, corn, barley, and oats in their whole forms.

Grains also contain compounds called phenolic acids, powerful antioxidants that help protect the body's DNA from carcinogens. Whole grains contain vitamin E, which protects cells from oxidative damage, helps prevent cancer and heart disease, and boosts the immune system.[9]

Possibly the most highly touted benefit of grain is its fiber content. In the early '70s, researchers began seriously to investigate the role of fiber in disease prevention. Scientists and medical professionals noted that the benefits of fiber are many and varied; high-fiber diets have been shown to prevent and treat a number of chronic diseases. A low-fat diet—meaning about 30 percent of daily calories from fat—in conjunction with increased fiber intake can substantially lower LDL-cholesterol levels. And the risk of colon or rectal cancer can be reduced by more than 30 percent by increasing daily fiber intake to 39 grams. Numerous epidemiological studies have backed up these findings.[10] Fiber can also ward off heart disease, fight obesity, and help control diabetes.[11]

THE WIDE WORLD OF GRAINS

Amaranth This ancient grain was a staple of the Aztecs and was revered as a life-giving, strengthening food. It's high in fiber and protein, and the protein quality of this superfood is superior to that of most grains.

Barley This small, round staple food was one of the first cultivated grains—it was planted in Asia as early as 7000 B.C. When the outer, inedible hulls of barley are removed, the remaining grain is nutritionally intact. Most barley, however, is further refined in a process called pearling, which removes the nutrient-dense layer. Buy the more nutritious "hulled whole," rather than "pearled," barley for hearty soups and stews.

Bulgur wheat Bulgur, a traditional food commonly used in Middle Eastern dishes, is made of wheat that has been steamed, dried, and cracked. It cooks quickly and makes a wonderful side dish seasoned with tamari and sprinkled with a handful of pumpkin seeds.

Buckwheat This edible fruit seed originated in Asia and comes from a plant that is closely related to rhubarb. In Europe, roasted buckwheat—known as kasha—is buckwheat's most popular form. A hearty grain that's high in protein, B vitamins, potassium, calcium, iron, and fiber, buckwheat can be used as a whole grain cereal or as a flour in baking (because of its low gluten content, buckwheat must be combined with wheat or other flours for baking breads).

Corn This tall, thick grass is the only cereal grain native to the American continents. As a grain, corn is generally used to make grits and other breakfast cereals, polenta, and breads. The variety of corn eaten as a vegetable is *sweet corn*, which is softer, moister, and sweeter than the grain varieties. Popcorn is yet another strain of the corn plant. Blue corn was originally grown by native peoples of the Southwest.

Couscous A traditional food of North Africa, couscous is made from ground semolina, the refined starch of durum wheat, which is mixed with water, steamed, and dried. The traditional variety of couscous is highly refined, but you can find whole-wheat, unrefined couscous as well.

Kamut This trendy grain is a type of wheat that has only been cultivated in the United States since 1978. "Kamut" is an ancient Egyptian word for wheat. Kamut is high in protein, magnesium, potassium, and zinc and is a good wheat substitute for allergy sufferers.

Millet This cereal grass is believed to have been the staple grain of the Chinese before rice achieved that status. A wide variety of millet is now grown throughout the world. It's gluten free and easy to digest. Boil it like rice, or cook it in soups and stews.

Oats Among the most recently cultivated cereal grasses, oats are a major grain crop in the United States, rivaling wheat and corn in production volume. Oats have a hard, inedible hull that must be removed before they can be eaten. The remaining grain, with its bran and germ layers intact, is known as the groat. Rolled oats are made by steaming, crushing, and drying the groats. Flatter, more finely rolled oat groats cook faster. Regular rolled oats are used to make oatmeal. Steel-cut oats are hulled groats that are sliced but not rolled.

Quinoa This tiny, disk-shaped seed (pronounced "keen-wah") is actually the fruit of an annual herb. This slightly ex-

---

The American Diabetes Association recommends a diet including 40 grams of fiber a day, especially soluble fiber, and the National Cancer Institute recommends incorporating 30 grams of fiber into the daily diet. In 1991, however, a study commissioned by the World Health Organization noted that the modern diet contains only one-third of the fiber intake of preceding generations and that Americans consume an average of only 12 to 15 grams of fiber a day. Yet fiber is surprisingly easy to incorporate into your diet: for instance, one slice of whole-grain bread has about 4 grams of fiber, nearly 15 percent of the recommended daily amount.

Go for the grains—make them about 50 percent of your daily diet. It's easier than it sounds. Start your day with a steaming bowl of oatmeal. Add rice, millet, barley, and other grains to soups and stews, and use quick-cooking bulgur wheat as a side dish or salad. If you're pressed for time,

otic member of the ancient grain family has been farmed in the Andes for about 3,000 years, and it was regarded as a sacred plant. Today, quinoa is again being cultivated in South America and to a lesser extent in the United States. It may be boiled like rice, used in soups and stews, or ground into flour for tortillas, breads, and biscuits. This ancient supergrain has about twice the protein of other grains and is a good source of calcium, iron, vitamin E, phosphorous, and some B vitamins.

Rice In the West, rice is usually hulled and then stripped of the outer brown layers—including the bran and germ, which contain most of the grain's nutrition—leaving only the carbohydrate endosperm. Whole brown rice is an excellent source of B vitamins, and contains calcium, phosphorous, vitamin E, iron, and fiber.

- *Long-grain brown rice.* The staple grain, with a nutty flavor and light, fluffy texture.
- *Medium-grain brown rice.* Slightly smaller and less elongated in size, with a softer, more moist texture than long-grain brown rice.
- *Short-grain brown rice.* The smallest grain, with the most minerals and a high concentration of gluten.
- *Sweet brown rice.* A faster-cooking rice with a sweet taste, sticky texture, and a high protein concentration.
- *Basmati.* An aromatic and flavorful rice grown primarily in India and Thailand. Also called "popcorn rice," for its distinctive aroma.
- *Kokuko, or rose rice.* A short-grained, sticky rice with a gelatinous texture. Also called "sushi rice."
- *Wild rice.* Not actually a "rice" at all, wild rice is a grass seed with a rich, nutty flavor. It is usually combined with other types of rices.

Rye Rye is a key grain in Europe, where it's a principle ingredient in pumpernickel bread. It's high in the amino acid lysine and contains B vitamins, iron, vitamin E, and protein. Use the flour to make hearty, nutritious breads.

Spelt This variety of wheat was first grown in Mesopotamia more than 9,000 years ago. When the Amish farmers immigrated to the United States, they brought spelt with them. Spelt, higher in protein and iron than other grains, is a good grain substitute for those with wheat allergies.

Triticale In the late 1800s, scientists experimenting with natural rye and wheat hybrids developed a seed-bearing strain now known as triticale. This nutty-flavored hybrid is higher in lysine and lower in gluten than wheat and is higher in protein than either wheat or rye. It's usually used in breads and baking mixes.

Wheat Wheat cultivation began in the Stone Age (between 8000 B.C. and 6000 B.C.) in Asia, and wheat has been the chief bread grain throughout the world for thousands of years. *Hard wheat* is higher in gluten and protein than soft wheat, and is used for making bread. *Soft wheat*, or pastry flour, is lighter in color and lower in gluten—and it's available in the whole-wheat variety. *Durum wheat* is used for making pasta, since it's able to hold its shape in cooking. Whole-wheat berries can be sprouted and used in salads or baked goods, or cooked to make a chewy, nutty cereal.

Wild rice This nutty, distinctive grain is actually the seed of a tall grass that grows in shallow waters in ponds and lakes. It has a chewy texture and nutty taste. Try combining it with regular brown rice for a surprising taste treat with lots of versatility.

remember that whole-grain noodles cook in a mere 8 to 10 minutes—less time than it takes to call out for Chinese.

CITRUS FRUITS

In the era of overseas colonization and exploration, sailors like Ferdinand Magellan and Christopher Columbus noticed that on long voyages at sea their crews were stricken by a curious and devastating disease whose symptoms included bleeding gums and the inability of wounds to heal. As it turned out, the lack of fresh fruits and vegetables aboard ship was the main reason for the sailors' development of this disease, which was later named "scurvy" and became understood as a vitamin C deficiency. Sailors began taking citrus fruits, especially lemons and limes, on long sea voyages; thus, more than 500 years ago, Europeans were eating citrus fruit as preventive medicine.

FIBER FACTS

Fiber is found only in plant foods; meat, fish, and dairy products contain *no* fiber, while whole grains have generous amounts. Fiber is crucial for effective digestion and elimination of waste products. Plant cells are surrounded by a wall of complex carbohydrates, including lectins, pectins, and starches, which are not assimilated by the body. Unlike fats, proteins, and simple carbohydrates, which are absorbed almost entirely in the small intestine, insoluble fiber is not digested and moves through the large intestine virtually unaltered, adding bulk to fecal matter and facilitating its rapid transit through the colon, thus inhibiting the formation of toxins and bacterial growth.

Two types of fiber are in plant materials, insoluble and soluble. Insoluble fiber doesn't dissolve in water and has a relatively fast transit time through the digestive system. Because it's bulky, insoluble fiber stimulates peristalsis, or the movement of intestinal muscles, which helps promote regularity. It is particularly effective for treating constipation and diverticulosis and may help reduce the risk of colon and rectal cancers.

Soluble fiber dissolves in water and passes through the digestive system much more slowly than insoluble fiber. It reduces cholesterol levels and blood lipids, helps stabilize blood sugar, speeds the excretion of bile acid (which can break down into carcinogens), reduces bacterial toxins in the intestines, and helps you feel full longer.

In the rinds and seeds of citrus fruits including lemons, grapefruit, and oranges are substances called limonoids, which stimulate the production of enzymes that can help deactivate carcinogens. A subclass of the broader class of phytochemicals called terpenes, limonoids appear to be most beneficial in lung disease and may also be important factors in preventing cancer. D-Limonene in particular is believed to help protect against cancer by detoxifying carcinogens in the liver.

Herbert Pierson, Ph.D., is a diet and cancer expert formerly with the NCI; he now heads Preventive Nutrition Consultants in Woodinville, Washington. Pierson has called citrus fruits a "total anticancer package" because of their high quantities of healthy phytochemicals. In fact, citrus fruits have been found to contain 58 known anti-cancer agents—more than in any other food. And they're a compelling testimonial to the value of whole foods as opposed to supplements: it appears that the phytochemicals in citrus fruits are much more effective in concert than they are as individual constituents; their health benefits are greatest when eaten whole, rather than as juice or in other extracted forms. One powerful antioxidant called glutathione is most prevalent in whole oranges, but when the juice is extracted from the fruit, it rapidly loses its glutathione concentrations.

Don't forget about vitamin C and fiber. Citrus fruits are packed with vitamin C. As for fiber, citrus fruits contain ample amounts of soluble fiber, complex carbohydrates—including lectins, pectins, and starches—which are not assimilated by the body. Grapefruit in particular contains a type of fiber called pectin in the membranes and juice sacs that helps reduce cholesterol.[12] Citrus fruits can also help prevent cataracts by virtue of their high content of vitamin C. A cataract occurs when proteins in the lens of the eye clump together and form a cloudy film, as a result of years of exposure to light and oxidative damage. Researchers at Tufts University Laboratory for Nutrition and Cataract Research found that vitamin C can help prevent the eyes from oxidative damage, since vitamin C concentrates 30 times more in the eyes than in the blood.[13]

Even though you're probably not worried about scurvy, the health benefits of citrus are too great to ignore. Fresh, juicy grapefruit is about as fast a breakfast food as there is. Citrus fruits make great snacks and healthy desserts. And as far as convenience goes, they're prepackaged and require no preparation—just peel and eat. What could be easier?

GREENS

If you think "greens" means a pile of lettuce drenched in dressing, you're not up to speed on the palatable possibilities of dark green, leafy vegetables.

Plain old salads are just the tip of the iceberg lettuce. And so many health benefits are derived from dark green leafies that you'll want to include them as a main factor in any healthy meal. They're loaded with carotenoids (especially beta-carotene), folic acid, and other nutrients. Greens with the highest carotenoid content include dandelion greens, kale, turnip greens, arugula, spinach, beet greens, and mustard greens. Other greens to try include Swiss chard, endive, collard greens, escarole, watercress, and parsley.

Studies have shown that greens are especially effective in preventing stomach cancer. At the First International Gastric Cancer Congress in Kyoto, Japan, researchers noted that a higher intake of yellow-green vegetables could cut the risk of gastric cancer in half.[14] The consumption of greens can also reduce heart disease, primarily because of the folic-acid content in greens. Folic acid helps to regulate blood levels of homocysteine, a naturally occurring amino acid in the body. At increased levels, homocysteine can become toxic and can contribute to the development of atherosclerosis and heart disease.[15]

One of the greens that offers a real nutritional jackpot is spinach. Lutein in spinach can help ward off cancer by enhancing the body's immune response—a mere cup of raw spinach or half a cup of cooked spinach a day may help cut the risk of lung cancer in half, even among smokers. Spinach may also help lower cholesterol levels, protect overall eye health, and reduce the risk of macular degeneration—the main cause of blindness in older Americans—by 45 percent.[16]

Most of the nutritional green giants are high in folic acid, which helps prevent heart disease and cancer. And don't forget about vitamin C, vitamin A, and fiber. One four-ounce serving of most greens supplies enough beta-carotene to meet the RDA for vitamin A, and four ounces of kale, arugula, mustard greens, or turnip greens supplies the RDA for vitamin C. Additionally, all greens are loaded with fiber, with kale, spinach, turnip greens, and mustard greens being the top contenders in the soluble-fiber category.

One word of caution: it may not be wise to rely on leafy greens for adequate vitamin A intake. Even though dark green, leafy vegetables are packed with carotenoids—precursors to vitamin A—the carotene in some of these veggies seems to have a low bioavailability, perhaps because the tough cellulose walls of the plants make it difficult for the body to assimilate the carotenoids.

Even if you're not on a quest for bigger biceps, graze on greens. Used raw in salads, lightly steamed as side dishes, or cooked into soups, stews, or casseroles, dark, leafy greens—available in astonishing variety—are potent protectors for your overall health.

The said unknown sickness began to spread itself amongst us at the strangest sort that was ever heard or seen; inasmuch that some did lose all their strength and could not stand upon their feet; then did their legs swell, their sinews shrunk and became black as coal. Others also their skins spotted with spots of blood, of a purple color. It ascended up their ankles, knees, thighs, shoulders, arms and neck. The mouth became stinking; their gums so rotten that the flesh came away to the roots of their teeth, which at last did fall out.

Jacques Cartier, writing in 1535 on the effects of scurvy among sailors; quoted in Harold M. Silverman, Joseph A. Romano, and Gary Elmer, *The Vitamin Book*, New York: Bantam, 1985

Red/Orange/Yellow Fruits

These colorful members of the plant kingdom contain a wealth of phytochemical compounds guaranteed to benefit your overall health and well being. The main compounds in red, orange, and yellow fruits—including strawberries, raspberries, red grapes, apricots, peaches, cantaloupes, watermelons, papayas, mangos, and red grapefruit—are carotenoids, which have been shown to decrease the risk of heart disease and many kinds of cancer, bolster the immune system, and offset macular degeneration, the main cause of blindness in older Americans. More than 600 carotenoids have been identified, and a number of these have been studied extensively for their health-enhancing benefits and potential to prevent disease.

Alpha-carotene seems particularly effective in protecting the body from the devastating effects of cellular damage, including skin, eye, liver, and lung diseases. Other carotenoids, including lutein, cryptoxanthin, and zeaxanthin, have also been shown to prevent certain types of cancer. In general, regular consumption of fruits (two to three servings a day) rich in carotenoids may reduce the risk of cancer by nearly 50 percent, slow the progression of cancer, and alleviate at least part of the damage done by smoking. Lycopene, another carotenoid, has been identified as an especially potent antioxidant, helping to protect the body from the ravages of time and preventing age-related illnesses, especially heart disease.[17]

One fruit that's been receiving top billing as a healing food is cranberry. For years, cranberry juice has been used as a folk remedy to relieve bladder and urinary-tract infections (UTIs). Scientists originally thought cranberry juice worked by one of two mechanisms: either by making the urine too acidic for bacteria to survive or by introducing hippuric acid, a natural antibiotic, into the bladder and kidneys. In the mid-1980s, the real reason for cranberry's efficacy in treating UTIs was recognized: a naturally occurring substance in cranberry juice prevents bacteria from adhering to the lining of the urinary tract.[18]

Some nutritionists, who note that the high content of sugar in commercial cranberry juice may offset any beneficial effects by encouraging the possible development of candida (yeast) infections, suggest treating UTIs only with pure, unsweetened cranberry juice from a natural-product store. Juice in this form is usually highly concentrated and admittedly not tasty; if you can't bring yourself to hold your nose and drink it, cranberry juice capsules are also available.

Fruits with the skins on also contain soluble fiber, in the form of pectin, which reduces cholesterol levels and blood lipids, helps stabilize blood sugar, speeds the excretion of bile acid (which can break down into carcinogens), and reduces bacterial toxins in the intestines. Most varieties supply between 10 and 25 percent of the daily need for fiber: in fact, guava fruit may lower blood cholesterol levels by as much as 10 percent, by virtue of its high fiber content. Fruits also contain ample amounts of vitamin C, as well as certain phenolic acids, substances that have been shown to prevent cancer by inhibiting cancer-cell growth, and flavonoids, which have been shown to help prevent heart disease and reduce cancer risk. Ellagic acid in grapes, raspberries, and strawberries may help prevent cancer.[19]

To use fruits in your diet, start your day off with a bowl of sliced peaches with whole-grain cereal or bread, snack on dried apricots, or add a taste of the tropics to your life with mangos and papayas. Fruits make great desserts, too: try a dish of juicy red strawberries or raspberries to end your meal. You may even lose the craving for double-fudge brownies and tiramisu over time.

RED/ORANGE/YELLOW VEGETABLES

An apple a day may not keep the doctor away—but four to five servings of red, orange, or yellow vegetables just might. An enormous variety of tasty veggies, including squash, yams, sweet potatoes, pumpkins, red peppers, and carrots, offer plenty of palatable meal possibilities and numerous health benefits.

The most well-researched benefit of veggies in the red-orange-yellow family focuses on carotenoids, those mighty phytochemicals that do everything from prevent heart disease and cancer to ward off the common cold. Vegetables with a deep red, orange, or yellow color have most of the same benefits attributed to members of the red, orange, and yellow fruit family. Foods rich in carotenoids have been linked to decreased risk of various cancers, including lung, colon, bladder, cervical, breast, and skin; lower rates of heart disease; decreased growth of cancer cells; enhanced immune function; decreased risk of cataracts and macular degeneration; and enhanced mental functioning.

Carotenoids have been shown in numerous studies to help prevent heart disease. In one 13-year-long study, researchers found a strong correlation between lower blood carotenoid concentrations and a higher rate of heart disease.[20] In this study, as in many others, the correlation between increased carotenoid consumption and decreased risk of disease was higher when all carotenoids, not just beta-carotene, were considered—yet another argument for consuming whole foods rather than isolated compounds in supplemental form.

Vegetables in the red-orange-yellow family also supply ample amounts of vitamin A, vitamin C, fiber, and other protective compounds, such as

FINDING FIBER

Several different types of fiber exist, and each form has its own properties and functions. For optimum health, fibers from each group should be included in the daily diet. But if you've been living on a diet of refined foods with few fresh vegetables and grains, go easy at first—incorporate fiber into your diet slowly to avoid possible gastrointestinal distress, such as cramping and gas.

- *Pectin.* Slows absorption of food after meals, helps lower cholesterol, reduces the risk of heart disease, and helps eliminate toxins from the body. Found mainly in vegetables, fruits, citrus fruits, and dried peas.
- *Cellulose.* Prevents hemorrhoids, varicose veins, constipation, colitis, and possibly colon cancer. Found in the outer layer of vegetables and fruits, as well as in some grains and nuts.
- *Hemicellulose.* Aids in weight loss, prevents constipation, lowers risk of colon cancer, and helps in removing carcinogens from the intestinal tract. Found in vegetables, fruits, and grains.
- *Lignin.* Lowers cholesterol, prevents gallstone formations, can help diabetics, and reduces the risk of colon cancer. Found in vegetables, fruits, and Brazil nuts.
- *Gums and mucilages.* Regulate glucose levels, lower cholesterol, and aid in removing toxins from the body. Found in grains, seeds, and beans.

Source: James F. Balch, M.D., and Phyllis A. Balch, C.N.C., Prescription for Nutritional Healing, *New York: Avery Publishing Group, 1990*

phenols and ellagic acid, which help to ward off cancer. In the landmark Nurses' Health Study, which followed 90,000 nurses over eight years, women with the highest concentrations of vitamin A in their diets had the lowest risk of breast cancer. Other research has found that stomach cancer rates are lower in populations that consume higher quantities of vegetables: in the Japan-Hawaii Cancer Study, the diets of Hawaiian men of Japanese ancestry were measured in 1968 and then reevaluated eighteen years later. Researchers found that high vegetable consumption helped prevent stomach cancer, possibly because of the fiber content of the vegetables. And vitamins A, C, and E and carotenoids lower the risk of cancer in general. One twelve-year-long study showed that lower blood levels of A, C, E, and carotenoids were related to a higher rate of death from cancer.[21]

All the evidence seems to point to a single, simple solution: eat more vegetables, especially those with deep red, orange, and yellow colors. Pile on the pumpkins and red peppers and carrots, as side dishes or in soups and salads. It's an easy—and delicious—way to ensure the most protective benefits for your overall health.

FISH

You've probably heard about the Eskimos' astonishingly low rates of heart disease, cancer, and other diseases: the media blitz in the mid-1980s relating the news of the extraordinary health benefits of the Eskimo diet led to one of the greatest health-food fads since oat bran. And the story is not a folk tale. Researchers are finding that the diet of the Eskimos, which centers on fish and seafood as the primary source of fat and protein, may be a nutritional model that can improve the quality of life of continental Americans, helping to protect against cancer, heart disease, arthritis, diabetes, colitis, gallstones, and other modern maladies.

Fish oils are packed with highly polyunsaturated omega-3 fatty acids, which have been associated with decreased incidence of stroke, as well as decreased risk of coronary-artery disease, probably by making the blood less likely to clot.[22] Omega-3 fatty acids also help lower blood pressure and reduce triglycerides (the major type of fat that circulates in the blood), decrease plasma levels of very low density lipoprotein (VLDL) cholesterol, increase vasodilatation (which, in turn, decreases blood pressure), and reduce the tendency of blood platelets to clump and adhere to blood-vessel walls—in other words, they're crucial in the prevention of heart disease.

Two compounds in fish oil, eicosapentaenoic acid (EPA) and docosahexaenoic acid (DHA)—polyunsaturated fatty acids—help prevent blood-platelet clumping and the buildup of plaque on the walls of the arteries, and studies have shown that levels of LDL cholesterol tend to *increase* with a decreased consumption of fish oils. EPA and DHA can help diminish the negative effects of a diet high in fat. EPA (at quantities of about 7 ounces of fish per day) can also help relieve migraine headaches and has been shown to relieve pain in people who suffer from rheumatoid arthritis.[23]

Omega-3 fatty acids may also inhibit breast-cancer progression and can prevent or slow the growth of cancer tumors in general. Additionally, diets high in omega-3 fatty acids may have beneficial effects against several types of malignant tumors.[24] The best sources for omega-3 fatty acids come from cold-water fish like salmon, bluefin, mackerel, sardines, and anchovies. Tuna, swordfish, rainbow trout, striped bass, oysters, and squid are also high in omega-3s.

But don't think that tuna-fish sandwiches with a hefty helping of mayo will help your heart. Total fat content appears to make a difference in overall heart health. One study found that men who consumed diets high in fish with a 30 percent fat ratio showed overall lower cholesterol levels, lower LDL (the bad cholesterol) levels, and decreased blood-fat levels, with increased HDL (the good cholesterol) levels. On the other hand, those who consumed a diet with 40 percent fat showed *increased* cholesterol levels. The study also found that one fish meal per day can significantly lower blood triglyceride levels and decrease the reduction in HDL cholesterol levels that generally occurs with low-fat diets.[25]

Researchers have found that a 50:50 balance of omega-3 and omega-6 fatty acids—found primarily in vegetable oils—is the best ratio. In the average diet, the ratio of omega-3s to omega-6s is about 1:10—a ratio that some experts say can be dangerous to overall health. When omega-6s are more prevalent in the body than omega-3s, they cause an overproduction of certain prostaglandins and leukotrienes, hormone-like substances that can decrease immune function, lead to atherosclerosis, form blood clots, and cause irregular heart rhythms. Consuming fish—especially cold-water fish like salmon or mackerel—about three times a week can dramatically increase the ratio of omega-3 fatty acids.

A note on supplemental forms of fish oils: megadoses of fish oil decrease the ability of blood to clot, which can be a serious concern if you're in an accident, require surgery, or are taking a prescription anticoagulant. Additionally, large doses of fish-oil supplements can cause stomach disorders. Prolonged, heavy consumption of fish-oil supplements can lead to a deficiency of vitamin E and can suppress immune function. In other words, the best way to get fish oil may be simply to eat fish. And doesn't a dish of poached salmon with field-greens salad or peppercorn mako with capers sound better than a gelatin fish-oil capsule anyway?

Nuts and Seeds

Nuts and seeds are packed with a variety of healthful compounds and can be a healthy and delicious addition to almost any diet—but that bit of advice doesn't give license to, well, go nuts. Eating bags of chocolate-covered almonds or downing handfuls of salted nuts at cocktail parties is obviously not sound nutritional advice. Because of their high fat content, nuts should be used carefully in most diets. But they definitely shouldn't be avoided.

Being a natural energy reserve for plants, nuts and seeds contain enough nutrients to fuel the growth of plants until they are mature enough to produce their own energy sources. As such, they're nutritional powerhouses, containing numerous compounds including protein, vitamin E, and fiber. Unfortunately, those energy reserves are stored in the form of fat, and the fat factor has given nuts a bad name—most nuts derive about 80 percent of their calories from fat. But adding nuts and seeds to the diet—sprinkled on breakfast cereals or added to pasta dishes—can be done in moderation: a one-ounce serving (usually about 15 to 30 nuts) contains between 150 and 200 calories—much less than a Snickers bar or a cream-filled doughnut. And the fat content of nuts and seeds varies widely:

- Chestnuts: 1.5 percent
- Sunflower seeds, pumpkin seeds, cashews, and sesame seeds: 40 to 50 percent
- Almonds, pistachios, and pine nuts: 55 percent
- Brazil nuts, walnuts, and filberts: 60 percent
- Macadamia nuts: 72 percent

Although nuts and seeds are relatively high in fat, most contain either polyunsaturated fats or monounsaturated fats, which may actually help decrease blood-cholesterol levels (certain saturated fats, found in animal products, are the bad guys). Nuts also contain essential fatty acids (EFAs), which play a crucial part in preventing cardiovascular disease, by virtue of their role in the transportation and metabolism of cholesterol and fats in the blood. The two EFAs are linoleic acid and alpha-linolenic acid. Linoleic acid is fairly common, while alpha-linolenic acid is harder to get in the diet since it's easily destroyed by processing. Diets rich in alpha-linolenic acid are associated with decreased risk of tumor formation and heart disease and can be converted by the body into EPA and DHA—types of omega-3 fatty acids. Alpha-linolenic acid is prevalent in linseed oil, walnuts, and rapeseed (used to make canola oil).

Table 4

FAT MAKEUP OF NUT AND SEED OILS

Almond	65 percent monounsaturated
	26 percent polyunsaturated
	9 percent saturated
Canola	60 percent monounsaturated
	34 percent polyunsaturated
	6 percent saturated
Peanut	51 percent monounsaturated
	30 percent polyunsaturated
	19 percent saturated
Safflower	13 percent monounsaturated
	79 percent polyunsaturated
	8 percent saturated
Sesame	46 percent monounsaturated
	41 percent polyunsaturated
	13 percent saturated
Sunflower	19 percent monounsaturated
	69 percent polyunsaturated
	12 percent saturated

EFAs also promote growth and are essential for healthy skin, hair, glands, mucus membranes, nerves, and arteries. They're important for regulation of cholesterol production, menstruation, and blood pressure, and for absorption of calcium and proper body lubrication. Inadequate intake of EFAs can cause or aggravate acne, dandruff, dry hair and skin, diarrhea, weak nails, allergies, and menstrual disorders. The best vegetable source for omega-3 EFAs in the diet is flaxseed—you can use it in oil form as a basis for salad dressing, and more and more natural bread manufacturers are including flaxseed in their baked goods.

Walnuts have been in the limelight ever since a study reported in 1993 in the *New England Journal of Medicine* showed that walnuts helped reduce serum lipids and lowered blood-cholesterol levels.[26] Other nuts have been getting their fair share of publicity: one study reported in the *American Journal of Clinical Nutrition* in May 1994 found that diets relying on almonds as the source of fat resulted in significantly lower cholesterol levels. Macadamia nuts, rich in monounsaturated fatty acids that have been shown to reduce the rate of stroke and high blood pressure, may also reduce LDL-cholesterol levels. Brazil nuts contain high quantities of selenium: a single Brazil nut meets the RDA for selenium, which can lower blood pressure, boost immunity, and inhibit the development of certain kinds of tumors.[27] And one study of more than 30,000 people found that those who consumed all kinds of nuts more than four times a week were 38 percent less likely to die from heart disease.[28]

Isoflavones, also found in nuts, are a member of the flavonoid family of phytochemicals and appear to have potent anticarcinogenic action. They act as antioxidants and help preserve vitamin C in the body. Ellagic acid is a type of phenol found in a number of fruits and vegetables, with particularly high concentrations in nuts. Its main benefit is in the prevention of cancer by impacting both the activation and the detoxification of potential carcinogens.[29]

Lignins, which may block or suppress the growth of cancer cells, occur in various quantities in many foods and are especially abundant in flaxseeds. Flax and other seeds are also high in omega-3 fatty acids, which help protect against colon cancer and heart disease.[30] Nuts and seeds are also high in vitamin E, which can inhibit cancers of the breast, colon, esophagus, lung, cervix, mouth, throat, colon, and stomach; prevent atherosclerosis and heart disease; enhance immune-system function; and slow the progression of nervous-system disorders, possibly offering protection against Alzheimer's.

Seeds have healing benefits of their own. Pumpkin seeds may help relieve enlargement of the prostate gland, and a one-ounce serving a day has been used as a folk remedy for this malady in many parts of the world. Pumpkin seeds contain high concentrations of certain amino acids that can reduce the symptoms of prostate enlargement.[31] According to Dr. James Duke, a botanist with the U.S. Department of Agriculture, about an ounce a day of sesame seeds, flaxseeds, and various nuts can also treat symptoms of swollen prostate gland.

So go ahead and go nuts—within reason. Add one to two servings of nuts and seeds (a serving is one to two tablespoons) to your diet every day, in the form of nut or seed oils, butters, and spreads; tossed into salads, stews, and stir-fries; or sprinkled on breakfast cereals.

BEANS AND LEGUMES

The little legume has taken on heroic virtues in light of recent research. Studies have shown that members of the legume family help prevent heart disease,

THE WIDE WORLD OF BEANS

Azuki (adzuki) These small, dark red beans, native to the Orient, are thought to be useful in treating kidney ailments and other ills. They're loaded with nutrients and are a good source of calcium, phosphorus, potassium, iron, and vitamin A.

Anasazi Similar to pinto beans, these red-and-white speckled beans were originally grown by Native Americans. Try them tossed with noodles as a cold side salad or mixed with rice or quinoa as a complement to any meal.

Black turtle These small, compact black beans are especially popular in Mexican and Southwestern cooking. Fresh cilantro, crushed garlic, and a little hot sauce are all you need to transform a pot of black beans into a distinctive side dish or quick lunch.

Black-eyed peas Also known as cow peas, black-eyed peas are a southern staple. They're rich in potassium and phosphorus and loaded with fiber. Try them the traditional way, served with steamed greens and a splash of vinegar.

Garbanzo (chickpeas) Garbanzo beans, or chickpeas, are a staple food in the Middle East and are high in potassium, calcium, iron, and vitamin A. These round, pale yellow legumes are traditionally used to make hummus—a thick mixture of chickpeas and tahini used as a dip or spread—and they're also great with grains.

Kidney beans These medium-sized red beans get their name from their distinctive shape. Kidney beans are a mainstay in Mexican meals, and they work equally well in soups and stews. Try mixing them with other cooked beans and tossing them in a light vinaigrette for a quick and easy, super-nutritious salad.

Lentils A member of the pea family, these small, disk-shaped seeds have been found in excavations dating from the Bronze Age. These little legumes are nutritional dynamos—they're high in calcium, magnesium, potassium, phosphorus, chlorine, sulfur, and vitamin A—and are available in brown, red, and green varieties.

Lima beans Lima beans have a distinctive flavor and are loaded with potassium, phosphorus, and vitamin A. They take a little longer to cook, but they're worth the wait. Serve them hot, tossed with fresh basil or rosemary and a little olive oil.

Mung beans These small, dark green beans are grown in India and the Orient. Sprouted, they are the mainstay of stir-fries and make a wonderful addition to salads. Try tossing a handful of sprouted mung beans in soups just before serving, or mix them with millet and a little ground cumin for a savory side dish.

Navy beans The hefty size and hearty texture of these flavorful white beans makes them the perfect bean for soups and stews. Or try mixing them with diced carrots and slivers of green pepper for a hot side dish or cold salad.

Split peas These flavorful members of the legume family come in both yellow and green varieties and make a wonderfully substantial soup that's easy to make and loaded with nutrients. Split peas also go well with nearly any grain and are especially delicious with buckwheat or wild rice.

Pinto beans Along with black turtle and kidney beans, pinto beans are a favorite from the Southwest. They're rich in calcium, potassium, and phosphorus, and they make great soups.

Soybeans The soybean has been a major source of food and oil in the Orient for thousands of years, but it was unknown in Europe and America until 1900. The soybean is the only legume that's a complete protein by itself, and it's the most versatile bean around—you'll find soybeans in a variety of forms, from dried or toasted soybeans to tofu, miso, tempeh, and tamari.

---

fight cancer, stabilize blood-sugar levels, lower cholesterol, and help prevent obesity. Maybe that's why bean consumption increased by almost 40 percent between 1989 and 1991 (according to the U.S. Department of Agriculture).

Beans and legumes are important in the prevention of heart disease, mainly because of their ability to lower cholesterol, especially LDL (the bad cholesterol), and reduce blood-lipid levels. By virtue of their high fiber content, a mere half cup of dry beans can lower cholesterol levels by almost 20 percent.[32]

Beans are loaded with both insoluble and soluble fiber. One cup of beans contains between 12 and 17 grams of fiber—as much as five large potatoes or four cups of corn, and enough to account for half the daily recommendation of 30 grams of fiber. The high-fiber content of legumes and beans helps control diabetes by slowing the amount and pace of sugar entering the bloodstream. Some studies have shown that beans can reduce the need for insulin by almost 40 percent, and eating beans can almost completely eliminate the need for insulin in people with non–insulin-dependent diabetes.[33] Research at Oxford University in England showed that a bean-rich diet helped control diabetes by lowering blood-sugar levels and improving the ratio of blood fat—an important consideration for diabetics, who are three to four times as likely to suffer heart attacks and strokes.

Table 5
LINING UP LEGUMES: CALORIES, FAT, AND FOLIC ACID

	CALORIES*	FAT (GRAMS)	FOLIC ACID**
Black turtle beans	114	.5	64
Garbanzos	143	1.4	40
Kidney beans	112	.5	57
Lima beans	108	.4	39
Navy beans	129	.5	64
Pinto beans	117	.4	73

*Per half-cup serving
**Percentage of RDA

Beans have also shown promise in protecting against cancer, including pancreatic cancer, and cancers of the colon, breast, and prostate.[34] Lignins, also called phytoestrogens, have been shown to have estrogen-like properties and to help regulate estrogen levels and activity. High consumption of foods rich in lignins may reduce the risk of certain types of cancer that are related to estrogen levels, especially breast cancer.[35] Lignins and isoflavonoids may also have a chemopreventive effect on cancers of the male reproductive system.[36] Other compounds in beans and legumes include phytates, which may help prevent certain types of intestinal cancer.[37]

Nature couldn't have invented a food closer to perfect than beans. They're high in protein, low in fat, cholesterol-free, low in sodium, and packed with beneficial nutrients that can do everything from reduce the risk of cancer and heart disease to stabilize blood-sugar levels. With some advance planning, they don't take long to cook, and the variety of colors, shapes, sizes, and flavors is remarkable. Try to eat at least half a cup of beans three to five times a week—cook up a big pot once a week and add them to soups, casseroles, and salads, or blend them with a little tahini or herbs and spices as a sandwich spread. And if you're afraid of a little gas, check the recipe section for gas-free bean-cooking tips.

ONIONS AND GARLIC

Members of the garlic and onion family have a long and distinguished history of healing. It is said that garlic was prescribed in ancient Egypt as a cure for headaches, throat problems, and weakness, and garlic has long been used in various cultures to treat ailments ranging from rheumatism, heart disease, and high blood pressure to septic poisoning and gangrene from battle wounds in World War II. Louis Pasteur recognized the antibiotic effects of garlic, and Albert Schweitzer used it to treat dysentery.[38]

Garlic contains more than 200 different compounds that have positive effects on disease prevention, including suppression of cancer-cell growth and prevention of heart disease. The so-called stinking rose as wonder drug has an impressive array of health benefits:[39]

- suppresses cholesterol production and lowers LDL levels, leaving HDL levels at normal levels
- reduces the tendency of the blood to clot and helps dissolve existing clots
- may reverse atherosclerosis
- blocks the ability of chemical cancer-causing agents to affect normal cells and may inhibit growth of already transformed cells
- stimulates immune function
- protects cells against oxidation

Organosulfur compounds occur in plants from the allium family, including onions, garlic, leeks, scallions, and shallots. Of the organosulfur compounds, diallyl disulfide, or DADS, may be the most potent agent in blocking or suppressing tumor growth.[40] Garlic and onions may also block the formation of nitrosamines, carcinogenic compounds created in the digestive tract. Epidemiological studies have shown that people who eat lots of garlic and onions have a lower risk of stomach cancer, probably by virtue of garlic's action in blocking nitrosamine formation.[41]

Studies of garlic indicate that the compound DADS shrinks colon tumors, and it may kill lung- and skin-cancer tumors. Another compound—called S-allyl-cysteine, or SAC—may lower the incidence of breast cancer. Garlic appears to work even better at preventing colon cancer when used in concert with an increased consumption of vegetables and fiber.[42] In high doses (about eight cloves per day), garlic can also lower blood-cholesterol levels by as much as 10 to 21 percent,[43] and it may significantly lower overall cholesterol levels and LDL levels while raising HDL levels.[44]

Garlic provides yet one more example of the benefits of whole food. Supplement manufacturers would have us believe that the key healing constituents of garlic are destroyed by cooking. But allicin—the chemical in garlic that gives it its pungent smell and the one that degrades readily in cooking and with exposure to oxygen—is not responsible for the health benefits of garlic. Additionally, the cost savings of fresh garlic versus supplements are substantial: a whole pound of garlic generally runs between only $1 and $2, compared to the cost of about $10 to $14 for just a quarter teaspoon of active ingredients in garlic supplements.

As for onions, these members of the allium family—including their relatives like shallots, scallions, chives, and leeks—have many of the same benefits of garlic. Called "the rose among roots" by Robert Louis Stevenson, the onion has been used in traditional folk medicine for years. Now, modern science is recognizing its many health benefits.

Onions help prevent thrombosis and lower high blood pressure. The juice from one yellow or white onion, taken once a day, can help raise HDL cholesterol levels by as much as 30 percent. Other studies by the National Cancer Institute have shown that onions may inhibit the growth of cancer cells, especially cells of the gastrointestinal tract and leukemia cells, possibly by virtue of their quantities of flavonoids, including quercetin, and their content of coumarin and ellagic acid. Onions also have been shown to lower blood sugar, prevent inflammatory responses, and reduce topical swelling.[45]

Pile on the garlic and onions in salad dressings, soups, and sauces. Experiment with all the varieties, from delicate shallots to more pungent leeks. And use them liberally.

The dynamic dozen is in no way meant to be a comprehensive list. It's simply meant to describe some of the more available foods and introduce you to their phytochemical constituents—to prevent you from throwing your hands up in despair and returning to a diet of Danishes and extra-cheese pizzas.

6

THE NEW ANTIOXIDANTS AND NOVEL COMPOUNDS

In a perfect world, taxis would be abundant on rainy afternoons in New York, the Sunday paper would always come on time, and the plethora of novel antioxidants and other healing compounds being recognized by scientists would be backed by a host of impeccable research. Unfortunately, the Sunday paper sometimes doesn't come until the pancakes are cold, and the research on novel healing compounds is as scarce as an open taxi at 5 P.M. on a rainy Manhattan holiday weekend.

Chapter 5 dealt with food as we know it, the cargo we carry home in paper bags from the local grocery store, the stuff we cook with and eat on a plate. Many of the novel compounds we're about to discuss are contained in standardized, concentrated extract form, in pills, powders, or potions at the health-food stores, and some are not as well researched as the food substances we've discussed. The "new antioxidants" and novel compounds are, in some cases, food, but they're not yet included in the average daily meal—unless you have bilberries for breakfast or formulate your salad dressings with blue-green algae.

Dozens of so-called novel antioxidants and healing compounds, from ashwangandha to zinc, are currently being researched, and many of the studies are seductive and compelling—but a complete discussion of all of these compounds would warrant a book in itself. So, on the advice of several experts, I've chosen what appear to be the top ten in this particular category, based on valid scientific research, promising studies and anecdotal evidence, and familiarity and availability to the average reader and consumer.

RED WINE

Red wine came into vogue in the late '80s and early '90s after researchers pointed out the seeming health benefits of occasional imbibing. Cabernet and Merlot rapidly replaced Chardonnay and white-wine spritzers on the cocktail-party circuit, and bottles of Burgundy saw all-time sales records, as the media played up the so-called French paradox. In spite of heavy consumption of cheeses and other animal fats—the French eat almost four times as much butter as Americans—the death rate from heart disease in France is 2.5 times lower than in the United States.[1]

The main substances of interest in red wine are flavonoids and polyphenols, also found in citrus fruits, onions, tea, and other foods, which appear to have a remarkable preventive effect against heart disease. Moderate red-wine consumption—two glasses a day for men, one for women—has been related to lower risk of heart disease. Numerous epidemiological studies have shown that light drinkers have less risk of heart problems and death from heart diseases than teetotalers.[2]

The exact mechanism of flavonoids' protective effect isn't known, but researchers postulate that substances in red wine can inhibit platelet clumping—the action by which blood cells stick together and form clots. The secret seems to be in the skin: white wines have very few flavonoids, while red wines, which are crushed with the skins on, are teeming with these beneficial compounds.

Phenolic compounds in red wine—including catechins, anthocyanins, and tannins—can prevent the oxidation of LDL cholesterol, thus inhibiting the likelihood of atherosclerosis. Two glasses of red wine a day may help inhibit LDL-cholesterol oxidation, offering heart-protective benefits.[3] A Kaiser Permanente study of 300,000 Californians found that among those who consumed alcohol, wine drinkers (especially red-wine drinkers) were at the lowest risk of heart disease.

Grape juice also contains flavonoids, but almost three times as much grape juice as red wine is required to reach the same heart-protective effects. The active substances in grapes include a compound called resveratrol, that shows promise in the prevention of heart disease. Resveratrol is a naturally occurring fungicide in grape skins that may help lower overall blood-cholesterol levels and increase HDL levels. Some research in Japan has shown that resveratrol prevents arteries from becoming clogged in animals.[4] And even though more grape juice is required to provide the same levels of beneficial components found in red wine, grape juice has a more standardized content of resveratrol; wines vary widely in their resveratrol content, depending on processing methods and types of wine.[5] Unfortunately, regular "table grapes" contain little resveratrol, since most grapes are treated with chemical agents to inhibit fungus and molds—thus, the grapes have little incentive to produce their own fungicides. Even organic grapes may be treated with natural fungicides that inhibit the grapes' production of resveratrol.

Along with studies that indicate heart-protective benefits specifically associated with red wine, clinical and epidemiological studies more generally have suggested that moderate consumption of any kind of alcohol can reduce the risk of heart disease, but consumption of wine and beer has been associated with a lower risk of heart disease than consumption of hard liquor.[6] Additionally, there is some suggestion that wine can destroy organisms that produce disease. Much of this is anecdotal evidence, but a few tests have shown that wine may kill bacteria that cause food poisoning, especially salmonella, staphylococcus, and *Escherichia (E.) coli*. According to Karl C. Klontz, M.D., an FDA researcher, even one alcoholic beverage with meals can reduce the chance of food poisoning. In one study examining people who contracted hepatitis by eating raw oysters, alcohol reduced the risk of developing hepatitis by 90 percent.[7]

Now for the bad news: before you settle down with a bottle of Burgundy and figure you're just appreciating a good heart medicine, you should know that high alcohol consumption—three or more drinks a day—is actually detrimental to heart health. Heavy drinking has been shown to increase the risk of high-blood-pressure, stroke, and other cardiovascular problems, and evidence exists to suggest that long-term, heavy drinking is harmful to the muscles of the heart. Some estimates suggest that heavy alcohol consumption causes 50 percent of cardiovascular disease, and as many as 30 percent of high-blood-pressure cases may be related to heavy drinking.[8] In the big picture, despite substantive evidence of the health benefits of moderate drinking—especially of red wine—you should keep two points in mind. First, the beneficial compounds in red wine may occur in other substances. Second, evidence shows that the consumption of alcohol has numerous deleterious effects that should not be ignored. In short, red wine can have substantial health benefits, but that doesn't give license to uninhibited imbibing. Moderate consumption of red wine—about three to five glasses a week, with meals—will likely yield the greatest health benefits.

MUSHROOMS

Long relegated to the realm of garnish or gratuitous inclusion in exotic entrées, mushrooms shouldn't be an afterthought to meals anymore. Research has shown that several of the more than 35,000 varieties of fungi have potent

- Red wine
- Mushrooms
- Ginger
- GLA (borage, black currant seed, evening primrose oil)
- Turmeric/curcumin/ curcuminoids
- Green tea
- Bilberry
- Green foods (spirulina and chlorophyll)
- *Ginkgo biloba*
- Co-Q 10

healing properties. So if you still think of mushrooms as only vehicles for baked crab and cheese or as decorations to drape on spinach salads, it's time for a change. Mushrooms, used liberally, can enhance almost any meal. Their rich flavor complements a variety of foods, and they contain glutamic acid—a natural substance similar to the flavor-enhancing compound monosodium glutamate (MSG).

Perhaps the best known of the medicinal mushrooms is the rich, flavorful shiitake, used in various oriental soups and stir-fry dishes. Shiitake mushrooms contain compounds that studies (by the Mushroom Research Institute of Japan and the National Cancer Center Research Institute in Tokyo) have shown to repress the growth of cancer cells, and compounds from the shiitake mushroom have been approved as an anti-cancer drug in Japan. Shiitakes also show promise as AIDS-fighting substances.

An anti-viral compound called lenitan in shiitakes may be responsible for the anti-cancer and AIDS-protection effects of shiitake mushrooms by boosting the immune system. Lenitan seems to have a role in increasing the production of interleukin-1 (a tumor-inhibiting compound) and enhancing the functions of macrophages and T-cells, the body's defense mechanisms. Shiitakes may have a cholesterol-lowering effect as well.[9] Some texts recommend 800 to 900 mg per day in a 4:1 extract form (one gram of extract is equivalent to four grams of dried shiitake) for general uses. For more therapeutic uses, 5 to 15 grams per day in a 4:1 extract form for several months has been suggested.

The maitake mushroom has lately been receiving much publicity, with promising research in such areas as AIDS prevention, cancer, and immune-function enhancement.[10] The maitake mushroom, also called "hen of the woods" and "dancing mushroom" in Japan, grows on the base of trees in small clusters and contains a number of beneficial compounds, including polysaccharides such as beta-glucan, which can stimulate the immune system.

Some promising research on maitake mushrooms indicates that they may help protect against high blood pressure, constipation, diabetes, and HIV.[11] Maitake mushrooms have also been shown to repress the growth of cancer cells in animals, and they show some promise in treating cancer in humans

Caution: raw mushrooms contain hydrazines, potentially toxic substances that have been shown to cause cancer in animals in large doses. Hydrazines are destroyed by cooking or drying—so if you're using fresh mushrooms, include them in cooked dishes. Another benefit to cooking them is that heat breaks down the fibrous cell walls of the mushrooms and makes some of the beneficial compounds more readily available to the body.

as well.[12] Using maitakes may allow a patient's dosage of chemotherapy to be reduced, while they support the immune system and mitigate unpleasant side effects of chemotherapy treatment.[13]

Perhaps the most promising research comes in the form of AIDS prevention. Studies in Japan have shown that trials conducted with AIDS patients and animals suggest that a substance called glucan from the maitake mushroom may help block HIV.[14] At the Japan National Institute of Health and the National Cancer Institute in the United States, experts suggested that maitake may be an effective defense against HIV. Other researchers report successfully treating Kaposi sarcoma with maitake extract.[15] For general use, 300 mg to 2 grams daily in supplement form is suggested. For therapeutic use, 25 to 35 grams per day has been recommended.

The reishi mushroom is a tonifying substance in the Orient, and this potent fungus has been used for centuries in China to strengthen internal organs, prevent kidney disease, strengthen the heart, protect against cancer, cleanse the blood, detoxify the liver, and increase overall vitality. Modern research has focused on possible anti-cancer effects from compounds called canthaxanthins (a type of carotenoid) in mushrooms and on treatment of allergies by a substance called lanostan which inhibits the release of histamines in the body.

Reishi mushrooms are also thought to promote adrenal function and enhance overall immunity, and they may be useful in treating diabetes and Chronic Fatigue Syndrome. Chinese practitioners maintain that the reishi mushroom helps to improve coronary-artery health, normalize blood pressure, relieve stress and fatigue, treat asthma, help prevent certain cancers, and treat a variety of degenerative diseases.[16] And reishi mushrooms are potent antioxidants that lower blood pressure and cholesterol levels.[17]

The new kid on the mushroom block—and one that's been surrounded by more than its fair share of media hype—is kombucha. This fad fungus is said to offer health benefits ranging from enhanced immunity and memory to decreased cholesterol and hemorrhoid relief. Kombucha, also called Japanese tea fungus, isn't a mushroom at all, but rather a cluster of bacteria and yeasts that is grown in a mixture of black tea and sugar for about a week, yielding a pungent, cider-like brew. Kombucha has been used for years in China and other countries, and while a sort of kombucha cult has grown in America, hard evidence of health benefits are mixed, with some promising research and some negative results.

The antibiotic activity claimed by kombucha fans may be due to its acidic nature, a direct result of the growing and fermenting process. Claims for curing cancer are wholly unsubstantiated. One study showed a mild anti-tumor effect, but it's possible that the results were attributable to the black or

It is well known in Japan that some types of medicinal mushrooms contain polysaccharide compounds which demonstrate anti-tumor activity.

Hiroaki Nanba, Ph.D., Kobe
Women's College of Pharmacy,
Japan

green tea—both of which have proven anti-cancer properties—in which the kombucha cultures were grown.[18]

Although the anecdotal evidence for kombucha's health benefits may be seductive, consumers should proceed with caution. Reports of gastrointestinal problems and liver damage from kombucha consumption have raised concerns among the medical community, and at least one death has been reported. Problems associated with kombucha may have resulted from the fermenting process: airborne molds, especially the highly toxic *Aspergillus*, can contaminate the kombucha culture if sterile procedures aren't followed, as sometimes happens when people choose to grow their own. Kombucha also has the potential for causing allergic reactions and interaction with certain medications. One of the most compelling areas of anecdotal evidence points toward kombucha's possible role in preventing AIDS, but even here, ironically, the opposite may be the case. Since the brew is made with a fungus and yeast, the health of AIDS patients may be compromised by a negative reaction of kombucha and yeast infections.

While the research isn't as conclusive as we might like, medicinal mushrooms do show promise as potent healing compounds. Shiitakes are easy to find and prepare, and their rich, beefy taste makes hearty soups and stews. Reishi and maitake mushrooms are harder to find in the produce department of most grocers, but are available in some oriental markets and at health-food stores in extract form.

GINGER

This spicy-sweet root has a long and illustrious history, dating back more than 5,000 years. As a key spice in trading, ginger helped grease the wheels of Middle Age commerce, and it has been used for thousands of years in the Orient to aid such maladies as stomach distress and cold symptoms. The ginger root has raised much attention among researchers who continue to investigate the possible health benefits of this ancient spice.

Best known for its effect on nausea, ginger has been shown to help ease the symptoms of motion sickness. In concentrated form, it may even be more effective than over-the-counter medications such as Dramamine.[19] Equally effective in treating motion sickness in car, boat, train, or plane travel, the herb worked for more than 90 percent of people in one study group. Ginger root also helped alleviate dizziness from traveling in as many as 50 percent of the people in another study.[20] Generally, the best results were seen with four 400-mg capsules of powdered ginger about half an hour before the start of the trip. For less severe symptoms, two capsules are usually enough.

Stomach flus can also be effectively treated with ginger: the best results are obtained with high doses in capsule form, taken at the first signs of flu symptoms. The generally agreed upon dose is four to six 400-mg capsules of powdered ginger taken at the first sign of symptoms, with regular doses as needed every half hour for the duration. Research has consistently verified the root's ability to mitigate the symptoms of colds and flu; it helps to suppress coughs, increase circulation, move phlegm, and treat low-grade fevers.[21] Ginger is also effective in treating female disorders, including premenstrual syndrome, irregular menses, cramps and nausea, and morning sickness during pregnancy.[22]

This versatile root has an astonishing variety of other uses: it has anti-fungal and anti-bacterial properties, and it has been shown to help eliminate parasites, reduce inflammation, treat asthma, prevent ulcers, increase energy and treat fatigue, reduce fever, help alleviate arthritis pain, mitigate the symptoms of most gastrointestinal disorders, alleviate headaches and migraines, and possibly lower cholesterol levels.[23]

Ginger may have a heart-protective effect by virtue of its ability to discourage platelet aggregation, or the tendency of blood cells to clump and cause clots or adhere to vessel walls.[24] Ginger's powerful antioxidant properties enhance its heart-protective effects, and Russian and Japanese studies have shown it to be an effective treatment for people with chronic heart conditions.[25]

While ginger in soups, sauces, and noodle dishes adds a pungent flavor and aroma, it may not be as effective as the root taken in different forms, mainly because it's difficult to ingest a therapeutic dose. The rule of thumb for therapeutic doses is to "use it till you taste it," says Daniel B. Mowrey, Ph.D., of the American Phytotherapy Research Laboratory in Salt Lake City, Utah. Ginger candy and crystallized ginger from health-food stores, ginger tea, ginger tinctures, and powdered ginger in capsule form are the best bets for natural relief of severe gastrointestinal disorders. But grating a little ginger into soups and sauces or sipping ginger tea can help gently calm the stomach, promote digestion, and add a potent zing to meals.

Gamma Linolenic Acid (GLA)

GLA is an omega-6 essential fatty acid found in evening primrose oil (EPO), black currant oil (BCO), and borage. Normally synthesized in the liver from dietary linoleic acid, GLA production is deficient in many people who consume large amounts of sugar, saturated fats from animal sources, and transfatty acids (such as those found in margarine, hydrogenated oils, and oils heated to high temperatures). The normal synthesis of GLA also requires a number of vitamin and mineral co-factors that may be missing from the average diet.

Omega-6 fatty acids are essential in a number of crucial bodily processes, including the production of prostaglandins (PG), hormone-like substances that regulate tissue functions and control every organ in the body. Since prostaglandins aren't stored in the body, EFAs are needed to maintain their production. Without becoming too technical, we could say that prostaglandins comprise a number of different types, including PG1, PG2, and PG3. The PG1 and PG3 series are the good guys, protecting the body against harmful occurrences such as high blood pressure, platelet aggregation, decreased immunity, and, to a lesser extent, inflammation and water retention. An overabundance of PG2's—converted from arachidonic acid, derived mainly from animal products—are responsible for many of these deleterious effects.[26]

The primary sources of GLA are EPO, BCO, and borage. Borage oil, produced from the seeds of the borage plant indigenous to the Mediterranean area, has the highest quantity of GLA. BCO, from the seeds of the European black currant, and EPO, extracted from the small seeds of the evening primrose plant, a native American wildflower, are also rich in GLA.

GLA has been dubbed a sort of wonder drug of the '90s. Numerous studies and clinical trials have demonstrated its ability to prevent hardening of the arteries, combat heart disease, encourage weight loss in the obese, lower cholesterol levels, decrease blood pressure, inhibit blood clotting, alleviate symptoms associated with diabetes, treat a number of neurological disorders, ward off ulcers, combat eczema, and ease the symptoms of arthritis and premenstrual syndrome. It's also a powerful antioxidant that's one of the key regulators of T-cell functions in the body.[27]

Some of the most compelling research on GLA is in the area of heart disease and cancer. In terms of heart health, GLA has been shown to lower blood pressure in numerous studies.[28] It also offers heart-protective benefits through its ability to reduce blood triglycerides (or fats), which are related to an increased risk of developing heart disease. GLA can also prevent blockage of arteries, thus reducing the risk of heart attack,[29] and EPO may lower overall cholesterol levels, reduce LDL-cholesterol levels, and decrease blood-triglyceride levels.[30]

GLA may even help prevent cancer, suppress the growth of malignant tumors, and selectively kill off existing cancer cells.[31] Human cancer cells can be destroyed by GLA, while normal cells are unaltered,[32] and GLA appears to be more effective at killing cancer cells than DHA, an unsaturated fatty acid found in fish oil.[33]

A dramatic reduction of gastric cancer risk has been found among people who consume large amounts of borages. In some parts of Spain, borage leaves and stems are consumed as a vegetable, and those people who consumed large quantities of borage showed a dramatic reduction in risk of gastric cancer.[34] EPO has been shown to kill tumor cells, and may help offset the deleterious effects of a high-fat diet, especially in breast-cancer cases.[35]

Numerous well-founded clinical trials and research studies have confirmed the effectiveness of GLA in a number of other areas, including mitigating the deleterious effects of aging, alleviating premenstrual syndrome, enhancing immunity, and treating alcoholism, asthma, diabetes, hyperactivity, multiple sclerosis, nervous-system disorders, rheumatoid arthritis, and eczema. Since it's unlikely you'll adopt the Spanish custom and start serving up side dishes of steamed borage, try using evening primrose oil, black currant oil, and borage supplements from the natural products store. General recommendations for supplement use include 500 to 1500 mg a day of borage oil, 100 to 200 mg a day of black currant oil, and 500 to 1500 mg per day of evening primrose oil.

TURMERIC

Known for its use in Ayurvedic medicine, this brilliant yellow spice traditionally used to make curry has a long and illustrious history. The root of the word, known as *haridra* in Sanskrit, has other synonyms that also denote the concept of night. The reference to night comes from a tradition in ancient India, in which married women applied turmeric to their cheeks at sunset, in anticipation of a nocturnal visit by the goddess Lakshmi.

The time-honored uses of turmeric in Ayurvedic medicine are broad and varied: it has been used as a stomach tonic and a blood purifier and to treat flatulence, liver disease, urinary tract infection, colds, ear infection, skin disease, parasites, bruises, sprains, cuts, wounds, inflammation, and chickenpox. Today, this bright yellow spice is used in commercial dyes, and it still has a role in disease prevention—including heart disease, cancer, high cholesterol levels, and arthritis. Some evidence also suggests that turmeric can aid in weight loss.

Turmeric owes its healing properties to active principles called curcuminoids, phenolic compounds that include curcumin (diferuloylmethane), demethoxycurcumin, and bisdemethoxycurcumin. Curcuminoids have strong antioxidant properties and have been shown to be potent anti-inflammatory agents, comparable in strength to many prescription medications. They can prevent the formation of free radicals and neutralize existing free radicals. Curcuminoids also have anti-viral, antibacterial, anti-fungal, and anti-parasitic properties and may help protect against cancer and heart disease.[36]

Curcumin, the most prevalent curcuminoid, has been shown to be remarkably effective in inhibiting lipid peroxidation,[37] and so consequently it shows great promise in preventing heart disease. Lipid-peroxide formation is a process in which free radicals are formed when oxygen reacts with fatty acids in cell membranes. Curcumin's efficacy in preventing lipid peroxidation has been shown to be eight times more powerful than vitamin E,[38] and curcumin has been shown to lower blood-cholesterol levels by almost 30 percent.[39] Curcumin can also inhibit platelet aggregation, a major causal factor in heart disease,[40] and it shows great promise in preventing cancer. Turmeric extract and curcuminoids have been shown in numerous studies to inhibit cancer growth and mutagenesis (damage to genetic material).[41]

Curcumin can protect the body against microbes and parasites[42] and is a powerful, natural anti-inflammatory agent that may dramatically reduce pain in people with rheumatoid arthritis and physical injuries. In supplement form, 100 mg with meals has been suggested for treatment of arthritis.[43]

The moral of the story? Learn to love curry. Make turmeric a part of your spice rack and your daily diet, incorporating it into a variety of dishes. Curcumin and curcuminoid extracts are also available in supplement form at health-food stores.

GREEN TEA

Maybe you've been imbibing chamomile and peppermint tea and eschewing "regular" tea, thinking that these herbal concoctions are somehow better for you. If so, think again. Dozens of studies of green and plain old black tea have found health benefits, ranging from reduced cancer risk to preventing heart disease, that far outweigh the benefits of herbal blends. Which is not to say that the herbal substitutes—not really "tea," in the truest sense of the word—aren't beneficial for certain, specific ailments. But they generally can't offer the often remarkable health benefits that black and green teas can.

In the simplest of terms, tea is tea is tea. All teas, excluding the herbal blends, come from the tea plant, *Camellia sinensis.* This brew is the most widely consumed beverage in the world, second only to water. There are essentially three types of tea—black, green, or oolong—but thousands of varieties exist within those categories, based on soil conditions, climate, altitude, and time and method of harvest. Additionally, the method of processing tea leaves determines the variety—black, green, or oolong—and has some effect on the amount and efficacy of antioxidants contained within. Green tea is the least processed: the leaves are quickly steamed just before packaging.

Green tea is of particular interest in the disease-prevention realm because of the potent healing compounds it has been shown to contain. Recent research has pointed out the efficacy of green tea in particular in preventing heart disease, lowering blood pressure, reducing cancer risk, regulating blood-sugar levels, warding off colds and flu, and preventing gum disease and cavities. But black tea may have many of the same benefits—it's just not as well researched, since Japanese and Chinese scientists had a head start in researching the benefits of this ubiquitous beverage.

Polyphenols, a member of the bioflavonoid family, are responsible for many of the healing benefits of green tea. Polyphenols in green tea are classified as catechins and have strong antioxidant properties. The most effective catechin in green tea in terms of health protection is epigallocatechin gallate (EGCG), which can be more than 200 times as powerful as vitamin E in protecting against free radicals. This powerful phytochemical has been shown to protect against digestive and respiratory infections, ward off cancer, reduce cholesterol, inhibit platelet aggregation, and inhibit bacterial growth. Some studies also show that green tea is an effective aid in preventing cavities. EGCG is a potent inhibitor of cancer and tumor growth in animals. Human studies have borne out the same findings: the National Cancer Center Research Institute in Tokyo found that death rates from cancer are significantly lower in certain regions of Japan where large quantities of green tea are consumed. Epicatechins are also present, but in smaller quantities, in black tea, although black tea has its fair share of antioxidants.

Quercetin, another important constituent of tea, has anti-inflammatory and anti-viral properties and can prevent and inhibit tumor growth. Quercetin works by preventing the release of histamine, a substance in the body that produces inflammatory reactions. It's also a potent antioxidant, protecting the body from the ravages of free radicals, and it inhibits the oxidation of LDL cholesterol, thereby helping to reduce the risk of atherosclerosis.[44]

In dozens of studies, tumors of the esophagus, colon, liver, pancreas, and mammary gland were inhibited by tea. Laboratory studies have consistently shown that tea can inhibit the formation and growth of tumors, mainly as a result of the polyphenolic compounds. These polyphenols are also thought to inhibit cancer by blocking the formation of nitrosamines—carcinogenic compounds created in the digestive tract—suppressing the action of potential carcinogens, and detoxifying carcinogens in the body.[45] In general, the amount of tea used in most studies was the human equivalent of two to four cups a day.

Green tea may also have some effect in offsetting some of the deleterious effects of smoking as well. Even though Japanese men smoke more cigarettes, the rate of death from lung cancer is significantly lower than that of American men, and one reason may be the high consumption of green tea common in Japan. In one study, smokers who drank no green tea had significantly higher rates of mutagenesis, but the rate of mutagenesis in smokers who did drink green tea was comparable to that of nonsmokers. The implication is that green tea has some sort of protective effect against lung cancer.[46]

One of the most compelling areas of research focuses on esophageal cancer, in part because there are few effective treatments for the disease. In one epidemiological study, people who were least likely to have cancer of the esophagus drank green tea regularly (one or more cups per week) and had a 60 percent lower risk of developing esophageal cancer than those who did not drink green tea.[47]

In terms of heart health, studies suggest that both black and green tea have potent heart-protective effects because they keep LDL-cholesterol levels in check. Tea may help reduce LDL-cholesterol oxidation and lower overall blood-cholesterol levels, as well as discourage the clumping of blood platelets, thereby reducing the risk of heart attack.[48] Additionally, increased consumption of green tea is associated with increased HDL-cholesterol levels.[49]

Both black and green tea may also control cavities and tooth decay, by virtue of their high levels of tannins, astringent substances with antibacterial and anti-viral powers. Researchers at Forsyth Dental Center in Boston found that tea was the most protective anti-cavity food they tested, blocking about 95 percent of the interaction between sugar and bacteria that causes cavities. Other studies have shown that tea may reduce cavity formation by up to 75 percent.[50] In supplement form, green-tea extract with 250 to 500 mg of EGCG content is the suggested dose for general use.

So have a spot of tea—but take it without milk, since the protein in milk can potentially bind to the antioxidants and render them unavailable to the body. Another tea rule: don't drink your tea scalding hot. In spite of the protective capacities of tea, people who drink tea at very hot temperatures demonstrate an increased risk for esophageal cancer. If you're worried about caffeine, set your mind at rest. Depending on the variety, tea generally has only a third or less of the caffeine of coffee. And to get the highest flavonoid concentrations out of your tea, use tea bags rather than loose leaves; the tea in bags is more finely crushed, allowing a greater surface area for flavonoids to dissolve into hot water. For the greatest health benefits, get over your coffee addiction and experiment with the wide and wonderful world of teas.

BILBERRY

Bilberries have been used for years in everything from jam to wine to dyes for clothing. Historically, this perennial shrub native to northern Europe,

North America, and Canada—a relative to the American blueberry—has been used to treat maladies ranging from lung disorders to diarrhea. The often-cited story of British fighter pilots in World War II who realized improved visual acuity in night-flying missions after eating bilberry jam may have some basis in fact—but use of *Vaccinium myrtilus* as a potent healing aid, especially for improved eyesight and protection against macular degeneration and other disorders of the eye, only began receiving serious attention in the 1990s. This potent antioxidant may also be an effective remedy against urinary tract infection, in ways similar to the cranberry. Additionally, bilberry may help prevent atherosclerosis, improve circulation, treat rheumatoid arthritis, and prevent gastrointestinal disorders including ulcers, nausea, and vomiting.

Bilberry owes its healing properties in part to its high concentrations of anthocyanins, members of the flavonoid family, including myrtillin, which lends bilberries their characteristic blue-purple hue and is a potent anti-bacterial agent. More than 15 different anthocyanins have been identified in bilberry. The health benefits of anthocyanins include antioxidant capacity, prevention of platelet aggregation and heart disease, and treatment of circulation disorders, varicose veins, and other diseases of the blood vessels.

The most highly publicized use of bilberry in modern times is in treating a variety of disorders of the eye, including glaucoma, cataracts, macular degeneration, night blindness, and nearsightedness.[51] Bilberry can prevent or treat glaucoma by virtue of its ability to enhance collagen and lower pressure in the eyeball, and it can dramatically halt the progression of cataracts, improve the ability to focus, and benefit overall eye health.[52]

Bilberries have also shown promise in strengthening the capillaries, maintaining their flexibility and preventing leakage, and allowing them to stretch and permit more blood to flow through. Capillary integrity is essential in preventing high blood pressure, diabetes, and atherosclerosis and in warding off bruising, varicose veins, numbness of the limbs, and increased susceptibility to cold. Bilberry is particularly effective in treating venous insufficiency (decreased circulation), especially in the lower extremities. Several studies have documented the ability of bilberry to increase the flexibility of capillaries, restore normal blood flow, and effectively treat the symptoms of varicose veins, reducing cramping, swelling, and numbness.[53]

Bilberry also shows some promise in preventing heart disease, primarily through the ability of flavonoids to decrease the risk of atherosclerosis and inhibit blood clotting, and by maintaining capillary integrity. Bilberry extract is commonly used in Europe as a cancer-preventive agent, and some studies have documented the effectiveness of bilberry in preventing ulcers caused by stress, excess stomach acids, or side effects of certain medications, primarily by increasing mucous secretions.[54] In supplement form, 80 mg of bilberry three times a day has been suggested. Or, if you can find it, try adding bilberry as a food to your daily diet—on toast, it's a great, healing way to start your day.

Green Foods

Much has been written of late about the power of green foods—spirulina, blue-green algae, green barley grass, alfalfa, chlorophyll, wheat grass, and more—yet in this seeming revolution, comparatively little scientific research exists. Anecdotal evidence abounds, however, and some promising studies have prompted scientists to begin more research on green foods. With ample scientific evidence, green foods may overcome their unfortunate reputation as a fringe food—what one scientist refers to as "pond scum."

Green foods owe most of their health-enhancing properties to their high concentrations of chlorophyll, the green pigment that supports the growth of plants. The molecular structure of chlorophyll is remarkably similar to that of hemoglobin, the protein pigment that makes blood red—the difference is that hemoglobin has an iron atom at its center, while chlorophyll has a magnesium atom.

The benefits of chlorophyll aren't a passing fad. As early as 1940, researchers noted the effectiveness of chlorophyll as a healing agent—treating conditions ranging from respiratory tract infection to cancerous lesions—in some 1,200 cases reviewed.[55] U.S. Army research showed that chlorophyll helped offset the effects of radiation: in a study of animals who were exposed to radiation, those who received a diet rich in chlorophyll lived twice as long as those who did not. Other research indicates that chlorophyll helps ward off colds, prevent inflammation, and treat inner-ear infections and that it is an effective agent for detoxification, deodorizing, and enhanced wound healing.[56]

Cereal grasses

Researchers began investigating the properties of the young green leaves of cereal plants in the late 1920s, and dehydrated cereal grass was probably the first multivitamin on the market, appearing on pharmacists' shelves in the late 1930s. The interest in cereal grasses began when a Kansas City food chemist named Charles Schnabel began to investigate what he termed "blood-building materials" to increase egg production in chickens. When cereal-grass extracts were added to poultry feed, egg production rose to 94 percent, and the eggs had significantly stronger shells. Other studies in the 1930s on milk production yielded similar results. Cereal grasses are rich in beta-carotene, vitamin C, and chlorophyll, with established antioxidant properties.[57]

Barley grass

The origins of barley date back to 5000 B.C., and the grain was being cultivated by the Swiss Lake Dwellers as early as 3000 B.C. Research suggests that barley-grass extract can relieve a variety of common conditions, including arthritis, asthma, skin problems, obesity, anemia, constipation, ulcers, impotence, high blood pressure, diabetes, heart disease, and kidney problems.[58] Barley grass is also an effective antioxidant, with high levels of beta-carotene and vitamins C and E. Barley grass shows great promise in treating gastrointestinal ailments by restoring the body's acid-alkaline balance.[59]

Japanese researchers have noted that when barley juice is added to injured cells, the cell's DNA rapidly repairs itself, a feat they attribute to a type of protein in barley juice with strong anti-inflammatory properties. It has also been suggested that barley-juice extract can promote the cell's ability to offset aging and prevent cancer. Barley leaves may act as effective chemopreventive agents,[60] and the proteins in barley grass can help remedy pancreatitis, stomach problems, dermatitis, inflammation in the oral cavity, and lacerations of the stomach and duodenum. Studies also report that barley grass is an effective treatment for arthritis and other inflammatory diseases.[61]

Wheat grass

Ann Wigmore, founder of the Hippocrates Health Institute, popularized the benefits of wheat grass in the 1960s and was its greatest proponent. She believed that rotting food in the intestine forms toxins that circulate through the body and cause cancer, and she recommended copious consumption of raw wheat-grass juice by oral ingestion and enemas. This brilliant green liquid extract from the immature wheat plant has been used for years as a blood cleanser, immune stimulator, and natural antibiotic and can be used even by people who are allergic to wheat.[62]

Some studies suggest that wheat grass can offset the harmful effects of radiation and pollution: one researcher, Dr. Ernst Krebs, Jr., claims that wheat grass is high in laetrile, a cancer-preventive compound.[63] Other researchers have hinted at the same, suggesting that wheat grass can decrease the ability of mutagens to cause cancer by as much as 99 percent.[64]

Chlorella

This microscopic, single-celled green algae contains more chlorophyll than any known plant and is a potent antioxidant. Studies have suggested that chlorella can bind heavy metals and other toxins and remove them from the body. Chlorella and chlorella growth factor (CGF)—a liquid extract from the nucleus of the chlorella cell—have shown promise in preventing cancer, enhancing the immune system, reducing heavy-metal toxicity, lowering blood pressure, and decreasing cholesterol levels. Japanese researchers have studied the ability of chlorella to protect against the harmful effects of radiation and to eliminate toxins, including cadmium and PCBs, from the body.[65]

Spirulina

Spirulina has been used to treat allergies, ulcers, heavy-metal toxicity, diabetes, liver disease, heart disease, and possibly cancer. Spirulina is rich in carotenoids, including beta-carotene, chlorophyll, phycocyanin—a blue pigment that can enhance immunity—and sulfolipids, which show some promise in protecting against the human immunodeficiency virus. The National Cancer Institute proclaimed sulfolipids "remarkably active" against HIV in test tubes. Spirulina is also rich in cancer-preventing phytochemicals, including chlorophyll, carotenoids, phycobilins, xanthophylls, and violaxanthins.

One of the biggest boosts to spirulina sales came after a 1993 report confirming the effectiveness of spirulina on children with radiation sickness, after the Chernobyl disaster. Spirulina has also been shown to boost immunity by increasing the number of macrophages, the body's defense against foreign invaders. Current studies are focusing on the efficacy of spirulina as an anti-bacterial agent. This potent antioxidant has shown promise in a few studies for a number of health benefits, including reduction of total cholesterol levels, increasing HDL-cholesterol levels, suppressing fatty accumulation in the liver, preventing tumor development, increasing immunity, protecting against kidney failure, and treating obesity.[66]

Alfalfa

Alfalfa's roots run deep—literally. Technically a legume and commonly used as animal fodder, this remarkable plant extends its roots as far as 20 feet into the earth and consequently is able to derive vast quantities of nutrients. The word "alfalfa" is originally from Arabic: centuries ago, Arabs began feeding their horses high-protein forage to increase their strength and speed, and the Arabic word for this green food means "the father of all foods."

Alfalfa has traditionally been used to treat ailments of the kidney, liver, prostate, reproductive organs, musculoskeletal system, and digestive system. In livestock research, alfalfa has been shown to help increase energy, prevent high blood pressure, protect against hemorrhaging, and enhance proper blood clotting. It's also used in treating stomach ailments, gas pains, ulcers, and poor appetite; it acts as a natural diuretic and laxative; and it can inhibit cholesterol levels, reduce tissue damage from X rays, control bleeding disorders, and possibly offer anti-tumor effects.[67]

Alfalfa contains high concentrations of the antioxidants beta-carotene and vitamins C and E, as well as xanthophylls and chlorophyll. Alfalfa also contains saponins, which have been shown to lower cholesterol levels, decrease intestinal absorption of cholesterol when taken before meals in concentrated forms, and (at very high doses) prevent atherosclerosis.[68]

GINKGO BILOBA

Ginkgo biloba became one of the wonder drugs of the '90s when considerable research validated its ability to improve mental function; it seems effectively to treat absentmindedness, difficulty in concentrating, loss of memory, and depression. The ginkgo (or maidenhair) tree—the oldest known tree on the planet, dating back 200 million years—draws its name from the Japanese *ginkyo;* in China, where it is widely grown, its name, *yinhsing,* means "silver apricot." *Biloba* refers to the leaves of the tree, which are divided into two characteristic lobes.

Seeds from the ginkgo tree have been used by Chinese herbalists for more than 5,000 years to treat coughs, asthma, and inflammations from allergies, and the leaves were used to "benefit the brain." More recently, ginkgo has been used in Europe for problems associated with impaired cerebral circulation. Ginkgo's most powerful effects are on the vascular system: studies show that it increases blood flow to the extremities and to the brain. Thus it improves memory, treats symptoms of senility, prevents blood clots, enhances circulation, and alleviates vertigo and ringing in the ears. Some research shows that ginkgo may reduce the tendency of platelets to clump together, thereby showing promise for treating heart disease and atherosclerosis. Additionally, ginkgo is a powerful antioxidant that may offset the symptoms of premature aging and may prevent cancer.

The main active compounds in ginkgo are flavonoids, including quercetin and proanthocyanidins, and terpenes, including ginkgolides and bilobalides—all potent antioxidants that are responsible for many of the beneficial effects of the herb. Other constituents, including ginkgolic acid and ginnol, can inhibit bacterial and fungal infections. Terpenes in ginkgo can also block the production of compounds in the body that cause bronchial constriction and increased mucous secretion; this would account for the plant's ability to inhibit allergies, asthma, and inflammation.[69]

Ginkgo has a remarkable effect on increasing circulation. In one study, ginkgo extract lowered blood pressure and dilated peripheral blood vessels, including capillaries. A later study also found that ginkgo positively affected cerebral blood flow in older patients, after a period of only 15 days.[70] One extremely painful result of poor circulation is a condition called intermittent claudication, in which the lower limbs become stiff and painful from a lack of blood after walking. In two studies, patients who took ginkgo for six months almost doubled the distance they could walk. Another study noted a 51 percent decrease in pain after only about a week of treatment with ginkgo.[71]

Another possible application of ginkgo is in the treatment of impotence. Since impotence is often caused by poor circulation, researchers examined the effects of ginkgo extract on impotent males in one 1989 study and found that 50 percent of the men studied regained potency after six months of treatment with only 60 mg per day of ginkgo—about half the amount generally used in studies.[72]

The strong effects of ginkgo on improving circulation may explain why such consistently positive results regarding brain function have been found. Poor circulation directly affects the function of the brain and can cause almost immediate symptoms, including confusion, difficulty concentrating, and fatigue.[73] In 1992, in the *British Journal of Clinical Pharmacology*, Jos Kleinjnen and Paul Knipschild reviewed 40 clinical trials since 1975 and reported positive results of ginkgo in treating mental function, with no negative symptoms or side effects. Most studies have used a dosage of about 120 mg per day of ginkgo-leaf extract, for a period of four to six weeks.

Some of the results described in the 1992 report included the following:

- In one study of 96 older patients, those who were given ginkgo extract for three months showed more than a 50 percent improvement in memory, a 54 percent improvement in concentration, and a 65 percent reduction in headaches.
- More than 200 people were studied by the German Association of General Practitioners for 12 weeks, and the physicians determined that 71 percent of the group who received ginkgo improved in terms of mental function.
- A group of 67 patients with vertigo, tinnitus (ringing in the ears), headaches, nausea, and hearing loss showed almost a 50 percent improvement after taking ginkgo for three months.

The same two authors also reported that 12 distinct symptoms related to cerebral insufficiency were relieved by ginkgo at doses from 120 to 200 mg per day and that the herb may work by preventing free-radical damage and lipid peroxidation. The symptoms included:[74]

- difficulty in concentrating
- loss of memory
- absentmindedness
- confusion
- lack of energy
- tiredness
- decreased physical performance
- depression
- anxiety
- dizziness
- tinnitus
- headache

Because of the positive effects of ginkgo on mental function, some rather extravagant claims regarding the cure of Alzheimer's disease have been attributed to the herb. But most researchers are quick to point out that that's an extrapolation they're not ready to make. Studies on ginkgo's role in preventing or curing Alzheimer's are currently being conducted, but the jury's still out. In the meantime, the best advice for protecting your brain may be to take the 120 mg used in most studies.

Co-Q 10

Coenzyme Q10, better known as co-Q 10, is a compound synthesized by the body's cells, a fat-soluble antioxidant found in the mitochondria. It is essential for converting food into energy, protecting the body against the ravages of free radicals, and strengthening cell membranes. Also known as ubiquinone, co-Q 10 is similar in molecular structure to vitamin E. The body is equipped to manufacture co-Q 10, but because of the complex pathway of delivery and the necessity for adequate amounts of other nutrients, some researchers feel that many people are deficient in this essential nutrient. Additionally, the ability to synthesize ubiquinone decreases with age—production often declines as early as the age of 20—and increased dependence on food sources may be necessary. The best sources are fresh, unprocessed foods, especially meat, fish (mackerel, salmon, and sardines), nuts, seed oils, corn oil, and other oils.

Co-Q 10 shows much promise in preventing free-radical damage from insufficient oxygen intake and congestive heart failure. It's also been shown to confer a number of heart-protective benefits, including treatment of angina (chest pains), and it can help treat muscle-weakening disease such as muscular dystrophy and boost immunity. Additionally, co-Q 10 can help recycle the vitamin E that gets used up in scavenging free radicals and can help prevent the oxidation of LDL cholesterol by free radicals.[75]

Perhaps the greatest benefit of co-Q 10 is in its role as a well-recognized antioxidant, offering the benefits of other antioxidants. Diseases caused by free-radical reactions include atherosclerosis, cancer, inflammatory joint disease, asthma, diabetes, senile dementia, and degenerative disease. Some researchers point to co-Q 10 and other antioxidants as potent defenders against these degenerative diseases.[76] Other uses of co-Q 10 include treatment of allergies, respiratory disease, declining mental function, aging, obesity, candida, and periodontal disease.[77]

Co-Q 10 has shown promise in preventing or treating heart disease, probably by virtue of its antioxidant capacity. The compound is highly concentrated in heart-muscle cells, which may account for the fact that deficiencies in co-Q 10 are most obvious in those with heart disorders. Co-Q 10 prevents oxidation of LDL, which can lead to atherosclerosis, more efficiently than does vitamin E or beta-carotene. Some researchers believe that many cases of heart disease and heart failure reflect a deficiency of co-Q 10. In one study, heart-disease patients had 25 percent less co-Q 10 in their blood, and serious co-Q 10 deficiencies were found in the heart tissue of 75 percent of heart-disease patients. Additionally, co-Q 10 can help lower blood pressure: one study showed that 225 mg of co-Q 10 per day reduced blood pressure in 85 percent of the cases studied.[78] Other research has borne out these postulations.[79]

Other promising but preliminary findings have focused on treatment of cancer. Co-Q 10 was shown to treat cancer, especially breast cancer, at dosage levels of 390 mg of co-Q 10 per day over a period of three to five years, and researchers noted a complete regression of cancer in the liver.[80] Some researchers have claimed that co-Q 10 is protective against AIDS, again by virtue of its antioxidant abilities. Since AIDS is an immunodeficiency disease, any compound that boosts immunity—including antioxidants—could theoretically hold some of the symptoms at bay. Co-Q 10 may also successfully treat muscle-weakening disease, including muscular dystrophy.[81]

How much is enough? The generally recommended dose of co-Q 10 is 30 mg a day for healthy people, but those with signs of disease may need higher doses—up to 150 mg a day. Some studies have shown that doses of up to 240 mg a day are safe and effective—at higher levels, the doses are generally divided into two doses twice a day, but since co-Q 10 appears to remain in the blood for long periods of time, taking higher levels at one time may be just as safe and effective. The best advice, then, is to make sure you consume enough vitamin E, which stimulates the production of co-Q 10, regularly eat fish like mackerel, salmon, and sardines, eat nuts, seed oils, and corn oils, and take a co-Q 10 supplement daily depending on your state of health.

CONCLUSION

Surprisingly little agreement exists on even the most basic of information in the field of functional foods, and much of the research is contradictory and confusing. Consequently, a neat and tidy conclusion seems a fool's errand at best. Suffice it to say that dozens of experts and hundreds of studies point to the fact that food contains healing compounds, but the exact amount and function of those compounds is not yet thoroughly understood.

If I had to choose between a diet rich in fruits, vegetables, grains, and legumes—with no supplementation of vitamins or other compounds—or a heavily supplemented regimen—with careless planning of food content—I'd take door number one any day of the week. But that's not a choice that must be made. The safest, sanest, most satisfying approach to complete nutrition is to simply eat a healthy diet, focusing on foods that are known to be rich in healing compounds, and use supplements when necessary. And remember that hundreds of epidemiological studies conducted on diet have come to the same conclusion: meals really do seem to heal.

PART TWO

ℛECIPES

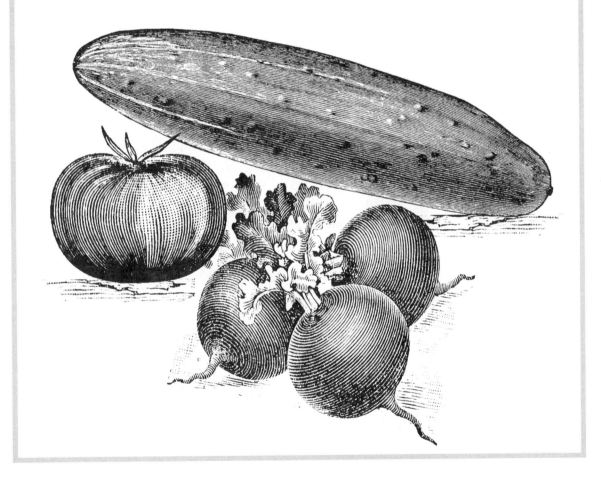

7

A FEW NOTES
ON PREPARATION

The following recipes are based on chapter 5's dynamic dozen"—those foods with the highest content of phytochemicals and antioxidant vitamins. But this is by no means just an attempt to coax some modicum of pleasure out of a gratuitous notion of nutraceuticals. On the contrary, the recipes herein can stand on their own, nutrition—with all due respect—aside. They're stimulating and satisfying, often gourmet renditions—and they just happen to be extraordinarily healthy as well.

In keeping with the recognized dangers and deleterious effects of animal protein, all of the recipes are dairy-free and meat-free, and no animal products are used, with the obvious exception of the fish dishes. All of the dishes are easy to make, are (of course) high in nutrition, and are low in fat. (One quick note on fats and oils: we're not talking about fat-free recipes. Many phytochemicals and antioxidant vitamins are fat soluble, so a modicum of oils is needed for maximum absorption and availability. This does not mean deep-frying your carrots—it simply means that a little olive oil on your pasta is okay.) And they're all based on the maxim that meals truly can heal.

Herbs and Other Substitutes

The following recipes use a wide variety of fresh herbs, which are vastly superior in taste and nutrition to the dried variety, whose volatile oils are often lost due to improper storage and handling. If you simply cannot find the fresh herbs called for and must use dried herbs, use one-third the amount. Purchase them in small quantities and store them in air-tight containers in a dark cupboard. Low-fat or fat-free soy milk may be used in the recipes calling for light coconut milk—either as a complete substitution or half and half—but expect a decided difference in taste.

Other substitutions may be necessary: if you can't find wild mushrooms or shiitakes, button mushrooms may be used. Try to find more mature button mushrooms (the cap has pulled away from the stem, but the top is still smooth and firm) for a richer flavor. If fresh shiitakes aren't available, the dried variety may be used—reconstitute them in just enough warm water to cover, and drain thoroughly. Frozen peas may be used instead of fresh peas—thaw them first and drain well. If fresh tomatoes aren't available, or if you can only find pale pink renditions of the rich red tomato, canned tomatoes are preferable. Buy the organic variety at your health-food store for the best appearance and flavor.

COOKING BEANS AND LEGUMES

Legumes include peas, a wide variety of beans, and peanuts. They're rich in vitamins, minerals, and protein, are low in fat, and are a good source of calcium, iron, and B vitamins. They're also surprisingly low in calories: lentils and kidney beans have only about 100 calories per $\frac{1}{2}$ cup serving and less than 1 gram of fat. And legumes contain none of the saturated fat or cholesterol found in animal foods. When sprouted, beans and legumes add valuable enzymes to the daily diet.

Because beans can be difficult to digest, there are some specific cooking and preparation techniques that should be followed to maximize nutritional value and digestibility. Beans contain certain carbohydrates that pass undigested into the lower intestine and are fermented by bacteria, thus producing gas. Before cooking, wash them thoroughly and soak them overnight to speed cooking time and make them more digestible. Discard the soaking water before cooking, since the water will contain the indigestible sugars. And if you're not used to eating lots of beans, make sure you start slowly, giving your body time to adjust.

To cook beans, after discarding the soaking water, rinse them thoroughly and add about 1 cup of beans to 4 cups of water in a heavy-bottomed pot. Bring the beans to a boil, cover and reduce heat to low, and cook until tender. The length of cooking time varies widely depending on the type of bean used—lentils, for example, are ready in about half an hour, while garbanzos and soybeans need to simmer as long as four hours (see Table 6 for exact cooking times). When beans are nearly done, add a teaspoon of unrefined sea salt and serve. Don't add salt to the cooking water—it makes the beans tough.

If you're in a big hurry, canned beans may be used—but make sure you buy the highest quality varieties from health-food stores. Better yet, rather than resorting to canned beans, make more than you need whenever you cook beans, and refrigerate or freeze them for later use.

Table 6

COOKING TIMES FOR BEANS

BEAN	COOKING TIME (FOR SOAKED BEANS)
Azuki (adzuki)	1 to 1 ½ hours
Anasazi	1 hour
Black (turtle)	1 ½ hours
Black-eyed peas	45 minutes (soaking not required)
Fava	3 hours
Garbanzo (chickpea)	3 to 4 hours
Great Northern	1 hour
Kidney	1 to 1 ½ hours
Lentils	30 to 45 minutes (soaking not required)
Lima	1 to 1 ½ hours
Mung	45 minutes to an hour (soaking not required)
Navy	1 ½ to 2 hours
Peas (dried, split)	45 minutes (soaking not required)
Pinto	1 ½ hours
Red	1 ½ hours
Soybean	3 to 4 hours

COOKING GRAINS

Forget about pressure cookers and all the complicated, convoluted recipes you've read for cooking grains. All you really need is a big pot with a tight-fitting lid, a pinch of salt, and a few cups of water. Rinse grains just before cooking, then combine about one part grain with two to four parts water—depending on the grain—in a heavy pan. Add a pinch of unrefined sea salt, boil the grain for 5 to 10 minutes, lower the heat, and cover and simmer for 20 to 40 minutes (see Table 7 for exact cooking times and amount of water). Most grains may also be soaked to shorten the cooking time or toasted first to enhance their natural nutty flavor. Cook extra for quick leftover meals and second-day salads and try combining longer-cooking grains, like barley and wild rice, or shorter-cooking grains, like millet and quinoa for an interesting combination of textures and tastes.

Table 7

COOKING TIMES FOR GRAINS

GRAIN	WATER:GRAIN	COOKING TIME
Amaranth	3:1	25 minutes
Barley	3:1	1 hour
Brown rice	2:1	30 to 40 minutes
Bulgur	2:1	15 minutes
Corn grits	3:1	15 to 20 minutes
Couscous	1:1	15 minutes
Millet	2:1	20 to 25 minutes
Oats	2:1	15 to 25 minutes
Quinoa	2:1	15 to 20 minutes
Roasted buckwheat	2:1	20 to 25 minutes
Wild rice	4:1	1 hour
Wheat berries	2:1	45 minutes

8

TOMATOES

**PHYTOCHEMICALS
IN TOMATOES**

vitamin C

vitamin A

glutathione

p-coumaric acid

chlorogenic acid

carotenoids (including lycopene)

San Francisco Cioppino

Serves 4 to 6

This light fish stew, with its undertones of basil and sherry, makes a complete meal when served with hot San Francisco sourdough bread and a bitter greens salad.

2 tablespoons olive oil
$1/2$ cup chopped yellow onion
$1/2$ cup finely sliced leek
2 medium carrots, sliced
1 small green pepper, chopped
1 cup sliced button mushrooms
1 clove garlic, minced
$1/2$ teaspoon sea salt
$1/2$ teaspoon white pepper
$1/4$ cup finely chopped basil
$1/2$ pound Roma tomatoes, chopped
1 teaspoon honey
$1/2$ cup sherry
$1/2$ pound sea bass
1 cup white wine
$1/4$ pound medium shrimp, peeled (reserve shells)
$1/4$ pound scallops
$1/2$ pound clams, with shells

1. Heat 1 tablespoon of the olive oil in a large saucepan. Sauté onion, leeks, carrots, green pepper, mushrooms, garlic, salt, and pepper until mushrooms are limp.

2. Add basil, tomatoes, honey, and sherry, and simmer for half an hour.

3. While sauce is cooking, heat the remaining 1 tablespoon of olive oil in a large, heavy skillet. Add sea bass and wine, and simmer until just cooked. Remove sea bass and set aside. Add shrimp, shrimp shells, scallops, and clams, and simmer about 10 minutes, or until shrimp is opaque.

4. Remove shrimp shells from wine broth, add sea bass, and stir fish mixture into tomato broth. Heat through and garnish with basil.

Sicilian Tomato Salad

Serves 4

This heart-conscious take on the traditional Buffalo mozzarella tomato salad uses mozzarella-style soy cheese and less oil for a lighter, healthier dish.

1 pound Roma tomatoes, sliced
$1/2$ pound mozzarella-style soy cheese, cut into $1/2$-inch cubes
$1/2$ cup black olives
1 small red onion, chopped
$1/2$ cup chopped basil
2 tablespoons olive oil
1 tablespoon balsamic vinegar
1 teaspoon honey
$1/2$ teaspoon sea salt
$1/4$ teaspoon black pepper

1. Mix tomatoes, soy cheese, olives, onion, and basil in a medium bowl.
2. Combine olive oil, vinegar, honey, salt, and pepper and drizzle over tomato mixture. Serve on a bed of field greens.

Tomato–Bean Salad with Parsley

Serves 4 to 6

This colorful combo of tomatoes, parsley, and beans is a fresh take on the traditional three-bean salad. Perfect for picnics and summer salads.

1 cup cooked pinto beans
1 cup cooked black beans
1 cup cooked garbanzo beans
1 cup chopped Roma tomatoes
$1/2$ cup coarsely chopped parsley
1 tablespoon lemon juice
1 tablespoon olive oil
$1/2$ teaspoon sea salt

Combine all ingredients. Chill thoroughly to allow flavors to blend. Serve on a bed of field greens or spinach.

Sherried Tomato Bisque
Serves 4

Dairy free and still delicious, this tomato bisque uses lots of basil and the sweet flavor of sherry to give a winning start to any meal.

2 pounds tomatoes, peeled and cut into chunks
1 $\frac{1}{2}$ cups vegetable stock
$\frac{1}{2}$ teaspoon sea salt
$\frac{1}{2}$ teaspoon white pepper
1 teaspoon honey
$\frac{1}{4}$ cup chopped basil (reserve whole sprigs for garnish)
1 8-ounce package silken tofu
$\frac{1}{2}$ cup soy milk
1 tablespoon safflower oil
1 tablespoon unbleached white flour
$\frac{1}{4}$ to $\frac{1}{2}$ cup sherry

1. Combine tomatoes, stock, salt, pepper, honey, and basil in a medium saucepan and bring to a boil. Reduce heat and simmer, covered, about half an hour.

2. While tomatoes are cooking, combine tofu and soy milk in a blender and purée until very smooth, adding water as needed to thin.

3. Press cooked tomatoes in stock through a sieve to remove seeds and basil leaves.

4. In a large saucepan, heat oil and slowly stir in flour. Cook for 1 to 2 minutes, being careful not to brown. Slowly add tomato purée and tofu mixture, stirring constantly until smooth and warmed through.

5. Just before serving, stir in sherry and garnish with basil.

Veggie Medley Tomato Sauce
Serves 8

Lots of fresh herbs and vegetables combine with ripe Roma tomatoes to make this a hearty, low-fat sauce that complements almost any dish.

2 tablespoons olive oil
1 clove garlic, minced
1 small onion, minced
1 cup chopped mushrooms
$1/2$ cup chopped carrots
1 cup chopped green peppers
$1/2$ cup chopped celery
1 teaspoon black pepper
$1/2$ teaspoon sea salt
2 pounds Roma tomatoes, peeled and finely chopped
$1/4$ cup finely chopped fresh basil
2 tablespoons finely chopped fresh oregano
2 tablespoons finely chopped fresh thyme
2 tablespoons finely chopped fresh rosemary

1. Heat oil in large saucepan and sauté garlic until fragrant. Add minced onion, mushrooms, carrots, green peppers, celery, black pepper, and salt, and cook just until carrots are tender.

2. Stir in tomatoes and herbs, and simmer about 20 minutes. Serve hot over pasta or Wild Mushroom Calzones (page 92).

Spicy Stuffed Tomatoes
Serves 4

Cumin, ginger, and chili peppers combine to make this spicy appetizer one serious hot tomato.

4 large tomatoes
2 tablespoons olive oil
1 small onion, minced
2 cloves garlic
$1/2$ cup chopped green chili peppers
1 teaspoon sea salt
1 teaspoon black pepper
$1/2$ teaspoon cayenne pepper
1 tablespoon freshly grated ginger
$1/2$ teaspoon ground cumin
$1/2$ cup cubed silken tofu
2 to 3 tablespoons pine nuts
1 cup cooked mashed potatoes or cauliflower

1. Wash tomatoes well and slice off tops. Set tops aside. Carefully scoop out pulp and set aside.
2. Heat olive oil in medium saucepan and sauté minced onion, garlic, chopped chili peppers, salt, black pepper, cayenne, ginger, cumin, and tofu. Add tomato pulp and cook for about 5 minutes. Stir in nuts and mashed potatoes or cauliflower.
3. Stuff tomatoes with filling and attach tops with toothpicks. Steam in a medium saucepan with a tight-fitting lid for about 10 minutes.

Wild Mushroom Calzones
Serves 6

Try this exotic, dairy-free take on the traditional calzone—with its wild mushroom medley and lots of rich tomato sauce, it's sure to please.

Crust:
1 package dry yeast
$^{1}/_{4}$ cup honey
1 cup warm water
3 cups whole-wheat flour
$^{1}/_{2}$ teaspoon sea salt

Filling:
1 tablespoon olive oil
1 medium red onion, thinly sliced
1 clove garlic, minced
1 cup sliced wild mushrooms (shiitakes, morels, chanterelles) or button
   mushrooms
2 cups shredded spinach
$^{1}/_{2}$ pound tomatoes, thinly sliced
1 $^{1}/_{2}$ cups Veggie Medley Tomato Sauce (page 90)
1 cup shredded mozzarella-style soy cheese

1. To make crust: combine yeast, honey, and water in medium bowl. Mix well and let sit for 10 minutes. Combine flour and salt in large bowl. Slowly stir in yeast mixture, mixing well. Turn onto a floured board and knead well (about 10 minutes). Place dough in a large, lightly oiled mixing bowl and allow to rise for 1 hour.

2. Preheat oven to 400°.

3. In large skillet, heat oil and sauté onion, garlic, and mushrooms until mushrooms are limp. Stir in spinach and tomatoes.

4. Divide dough into six equal pieces. Form into balls and roll out into 8-inch rounds. Spread each round with a few tablespoons of tomato sauce, then fill with mushroom mixture and sprinkle with cheese. Fold in half, moisten edges, and pinch to seal.

5. Arrange calzones in a lightly oiled casserole and bake at 400° for about 10 minutes, or until crust is browned. Cover with remaining tomato sauce and bake an additional 10 minutes.

Spanish Paella

Serves 4

This tasty Spanish dish combines brown and basmati rices with fresh vegetables and pungent spices. Serve as a main course with a tossed green salad.

$^1/_2$ cup long-grain brown rice
2 cups vegetable stock
$^1/_2$ cup basmati rice
1 tablespoon olive oil
1 large yellow onion, chopped
2 cloves garlic, minced
1 medium red pepper, chopped
1 medium green pepper, chopped
$^1/_2$ cup sliced button mushrooms
1 $^1/_2$ cups cubed eggplant
$^1/_2$ cup sliced black olives
1 teaspoon sea salt
$^1/_2$ teaspoon black pepper
$^1/_2$ teaspoon ground cumin
1 pound tomatoes, coarsely chopped

1. Combine brown rice and stock in large saucepan. Bring to boil, then reduce to simmer and cook, covered, about 10 minutes. Add basmati rice and cook for an additional 30 minutes.

2. Preheat oven to 400°.

3. While rice is cooking, heat oil in a large, oven-proof skillet and add chopped onion, garlic, red pepper, green pepper, mushrooms, eggplant, olives, salt, pepper, and cumin. Sauté until peppers are tender (about 5 minutes).

4. Stir tomatoes and rice mixture into vegetables and bake in 400° oven for about 10 minutes.

Cilantro Salsa
Serves 6 to 8

With the pungent flavors of cilantro and cumin, this version of a traditional pico de gallo is a tasty start to any Mexican food meal, or as a party dish all by itself.

3 cups chopped, very ripe tomatoes
1 medium Vidalia onion, finely chopped
1 large Anaheim chile, finely chopped
$1/2$ cup finely chopped cilantro
1 tablespoon ground cumin
2 tablespoons lime juice

Combine all ingredients and refrigerate to allow flavors to blend. Let warm to room temperature before serving, and serve with whole-grain chips and crudités.

Hot Gingered Tomatoes
Serves 4

Shiitake mushrooms, sesame oil, and ginger combine with luscious, ripe tomatoes for a wonderful side dish with a decidedly oriental flavor.

1 tablespoon toasted sesame oil
1 cup sliced shiitake mushrooms
1 bunch scallions, sliced, with green tops
$1/4$ cup freshly grated ginger
1 tablespoon tamari
1 tablespoon honey
2 teaspoons arrowroot
$1/2$ to 1 cup water
2 medium tomatoes, cut into quarters

1. Heat oil in medium skillet and sauté mushrooms, scallions, and ginger until mushrooms are limp. Stir in tamari and honey.

2. Dissolve arrowroot in water and add to skillet, mixing well. Cook for about 2 minutes, or until thick and bubbly. Add water as needed.

3. Add tomatoes and stir carefully, cooking until just done and well coated with glaze.

9

CRUCIFEROUS VEGETABLES

**PHYTOCHEMICALS
IN CRUCIFEROUS
VEGETABLES**

vitamin C

vitamin A

sulforaphane

indoles (including indole-3-carbinol)

folic acid

fiber

isothiocyanates

Broccoli and Pine-Nut Casserole
Serves 4 to 6

This creamy, dairy-free delight combines broccoli with the delicate taste of pine nuts and fresh sage for a quick and easy side dish.

$^1/_4$ cup pine nuts
2 pounds broccoli tops, cut into florets
1 8-ounce package silken tofu
1 teaspoon sea salt
$^1/_4$ teaspoon white pepper
1 cup grated soy cheese
1 tablespoon whole-wheat flour
$^1/_4$ cup finely chopped fresh sage
$^1/_4$ cup whole-wheat bread crumbs

1. Preheat oven to 375°.
2. Toast pine nuts at 375° for 5 minutes.
3. While nuts are toasting, steam broccoli just until bright green but still crunchy.
4. Combine tofu, salt, and pepper, and mix until creamy. Add soy cheese, flour, sage, bread crumbs, and half of the pine nuts.
5. Add broccoli to tofu mixture and mix well. Turn into lightly oiled casserole and sprinkle with remaining pine nuts. Bake at 375° about 15 minutes.

Indian Vegetable Curry
Serves 6

A truly traditional Indian recipe, this spicy concoction makes an intriguing party dish with its unexpected addition of raisins and apple. Serve with warmed pita bread and Collard and Carrot Raita (page 138).

1 tablespoon light sesame oil
1 cup diced onion
2 cloves garlic
1 teaspoon ground cumin
1 teaspoon sea salt
1 teaspoon black pepper
1 tablespoon dried curry blend
2 tablespoons fresh grated ginger
2 tablespoons whole-wheat flour
2 cups water
1 cup broccoli florets
1 cup cauliflower florets
$^1/_2$ cup chopped carrots
$^1/_2$ cup fresh green peas
$^1/_2$ cup diced apple
$^1/_2$ cup raisins
1 cup cubed firm tofu

1. Heat oil in a large skillet and sauté onion and garlic until golden. Add cumin, salt, pepper, curry, and ginger.

2. Stir in flour and cook 2 to 3 minutes. Slowly add water and mix until creamy and smooth.

3. Add broccoli, cauliflower, carrots, peas, apple, raisins, and tofu, and cook until mixture is thick and bubbly and vegetables are tender.

Brussels Sprouts with Honey–Ginger Glaze
Serves 4

So you don't think you like brussels sprouts? Try this sweet and tangy side dish—you'll be an instant convert!

1 ¹/₂ pounds brussels sprouts, halved, with stems removed
1 tablespoon olive oil
¹/₄ cup freshly grated ginger
¹/₂ teaspoon sea salt
¹/₂ cup grated carrot
2 tablespoons honey
1 tablespoon rice vinegar

1. Steam brussels sprouts for about 5 minutes, until just tender. Drain well.
2. While brussels sprouts are cooking, heat oil in large skillet and add ginger, salt, grated carrot, honey, and vinegar. Cook over medium heat until thick and bubbly.
3. Add cooked brussels sprouts, mixing well to coat thoroughly with glaze. Cook for 5 minutes longer until sprouts are very tender. Serve hot.

Smoky Shiitake–Brussels Sprouts Salad
Serves 4 to 6

A wonderful combination of pungent brussels sprouts and the slightly smoky flavor of shiitake mushrooms, complemented with crunchy toasted walnuts, makes this a memorable start to any meal.

¹/₄ cup chopped walnuts
2 pounds brussels sprouts, halved, with stems removed
1 tablespoon olive oil
¹/₂ cup sliced shiitake mushrooms
1 small red onion, sliced
¹/₂ teaspoon sea salt
1 teaspoon black pepper

1. Toast walnuts at 375° for about 8 to 10 minutes. Steam brussels sprouts for about 5 minutes, until just tender. Drain well.
2. While brussels sprouts are cooking, heat oil in large skillet and sauté mushrooms, onion, salt, and pepper.
3. Add cooked brussels sprouts to mushroom mixture. Stir in walnuts and chill thoroughly to allow flavors to blend. Serve on a bed of radicchio leaves.

Cauliflower Paratha
Serves 4 to 6

Try this tasty bread as a unique way to present cauliflower. Serve it with Indian Veg-etable Curry (page 97) for a decidedly different dinner meal.

2 cups whole-wheat flour
$1/2$ teaspoon sea salt
1 cup water
2 cups chopped cauliflower
$1/4$ cup celery
1 medium onion, diced
1 small green pepper, diced
1 cup mashed firm tofu
1 teaspoon sea salt
1 teaspoon black pepper
1 teaspoon cumin seed
1 teaspoon fennel seed
Safflower oil for frying

1. Combine flour, salt, and water, mixing well. Set aside for 15 minutes.

2. While dough is sitting, combine cauliflower, celery, onion, green pepper, tofu, and salt in medium pan and steam lightly, until cauliflower is tender. Drain and cool thoroughly. Stir in black pepper, cumin, and fennel, mixing well.

3. Knead dough lightly, divide it into 12 balls, and roll each ball out to about 5 inches in diameter. Fill each with cauliflower mixture and fold in half. Moisten the edges of the dough and press together. Flatten each lightly with the palm of your hand.

4. Heat oil in a heavy skillet and carefully slide each paratha into the skillet. Cook until both sides are golden. Drain on paper towels and serve hot.

Red and Green Cabbage Salad

Serves 6

A slightly exotic version of the traditional coleslaw, this fresh-tasting salad is the perfect start to a hearty soup meal, and makes a wonderful light lunch with bread.

1 small head red cabbage, grated
1 small head green cabbage, grated
$^1/_2$ cup raisins
2 tablespoons olive oil
2 tablespoons rice vinegar
2 tablespoons honey
$^1/_2$ teaspoon coarsely grated black pepper
1 teaspoon celery seed
$^1/_2$ teaspoon sea salt

Combine all ingredients and chill thoroughly to allow flavors to blend.

Broccoli–Cauliflower Bisque

Serves 4 to 6

This rich and creamy soup is dairy free and surprisingly low fat. Serve it as a first course, or as a light meal in itself with fresh, hot rolls and a crispy green salad.

1 tablespoon olive oil
1 small yellow onion, chopped
2 cloves garlic, minced
$^3/_4$ pound broccoli florets
$^1/_2$ pound cauliflower florets
$^1/_2$ teaspoon sea salt
1 teaspoon white pepper
3 cups vegetable stock
1 8-ounce package silken tofu
$^1/_2$ cup white wine or sherry
Parsley for garnish

1. Heat oil in large saucepan and sauté onion and garlic until golden.
2. Add broccoli, cauliflower, salt, and pepper, and sauté until broccoli is bright green. Stir in vegetable stock and simmer, covered, until broccoli and cauliflower are tender.
3. Purée broccoli mixture with tofu until very creamy. Return to pot, stir in wine or sherry, and warm through. Garnish with sprigs of parsley.

Wild Mushroom Cabbage Rolls

Serves 8

A quick and easy take on an Old World favorite, this dish uses a combination of wild mushrooms, pine nuts, and shallots for an exotic appetizer or a main course.

$^1/_2$ cup pine nuts
1 tablespoon olive oil
1 cup wild mushrooms (morels, chanterelles, porcini) or button mushrooms
$^1/_4$ cup chopped shallots
2 cloves garlic, minced
1 teaspoon sea salt
2 cups cooked brown rice
1 pound green cabbage

1. Toast pine nuts at 375° for 5 minutes.
2. Heat oil in a medium skillet and sauté mushrooms, shallots, garlic, and salt until mushrooms are limp. Stir in pine nuts and brown rice and let cool.
3. Wash individual leaves of cabbage, steam for 1 minute, and let cool.
4. Preheat oven to 375°.
5. Roll rice mixture up in 2 or 3 leaves of cabbage for each roll, and place each roll in lightly oiled glass casserole dish, seamside down. Cover lightly with foil and cook at 375° for 20 to 30 minutes.

Broccoli Rabe Stir-Fry
Serves 6

This dish uses broccoli rabe and chicory for an intriguing, slightly bitter variation on the traditional stir-fry. Serve over brown rice for a fast family meal.

1 tablespoon olive oil
$1/2$ cup sliced red onion
2 cloves garlic, minced
1 cup broccoli rabe, chopped
3 carrots, sliced on the diagonal
1 small red pepper, diced
1 teaspoon sea salt
$1/2$ teaspoon black pepper
1 cup cubed firm tofu
1 cup chicory, chopped
$1/2$ cup water
1 tablespoon arrowroot
2 tablespoons honey
2 tablespoons rice vinegar

1. Heat oil in a medium skillet. Sauté onion, garlic, broccoli, carrots, red pepper, salt, and black pepper until broccoli is tender.

2. Stir in tofu and chicory, and cook just until chicory begins to wilt.

3. In a small bowl, combine water, arrowroot, honey, and vinegar. Stir into vegetable and tofu mixture, and heat through until thick and bubbly.

Peppered Cabbage Stew

Serves 6 to 8

This hearty, healthy stew uses the traditional combination of cabbage, potatoes, and carrots with lots of black and red pepper for a winning, one-dish meal.

1 tablespoon olive oil
1 medium yellow onion, diced
1 clove garlic, minced
1 cup chopped carrots
$^1/_2$ cup chopped celery
1 cup diced red potatoes, with the skins on
$^1/_2$ teaspoon sea salt
1 teaspoon coarsely ground black pepper
$^1/_2$ teaspoon crushed red pepper flakes
4 cups vegetable stock
2 cups chopped green cabbage
$^1/_2$ cup cooked garbanzo or other beans

1. Heat oil in large pot and sauté onion and garlic until onion is translucent.
2. Add carrots, celery, potatoes, salt, black pepper, and red pepper, and cook until potatoes are tender.
3. Stir in stock, cabbage, and beans, and simmer until cabbage is tender (about 7 minutes).

10

SOYBEANS

PHYTOCHEMICALS
IN SOYBEANS

isoflavones

genistein

phytic acid

protease inhibitors

phytoestrogens

Spicy Tofu Dal

Serves 6

This spicy Indian dish is a one-pot meal in itself. Serve with whole-wheat pitas and a salad of chilled cucumbers, diced tomatoes, and chopped cilantro.

1 cup lentils
4 cups water
1 tablespoon safflower oil
1 medium yellow onion, diced
2 cloves garlic, minced
1 to 2 small jalapeno peppers, finely diced
1 cup cubed firm tofu
1 teaspoon sea salt
1 teaspoon white pepper
1 tablespoon ground cumin
2 tablespoons freshly grated ginger
1 large tomato, chopped
1 cup fresh green peas
Juice from 1 lemon
1 tablespoon cumin seeds

1. Combine lentils and water and cook for 30 minutes, or until tender.

2. While lentils are cooking, heat oil in medium skillet and sauté onion, garlic, diced jalapeno peppers, tofu, salt, white pepper, ground cumin, and ginger. Cook until onions are soft and tofu is lightly browned.

3. Add chopped tomato, peas, and lemon juice to the vegetables and cook until peas are tender. Add to lentils and garnish with cumin seeds.

Burritos Grande

Serves 8

Try this spicy, dairy-free take on traditional burritos. They're loaded with lots of low-fat protein—a perfect transitional food for first-time vegetarians.

1 tablespoon canola oil
1 large yellow onion, chopped
1 medium green pepper, diced
$1/2$ cup sliced button mushrooms
1 cup cubed firm tofu
1 teaspoon sea salt
1 tablespoon chili powder
$1/2$ teaspoon cayenne
1 teaspoon ground cumin
$1/2$ teaspoon black pepper
4 cups cooked black beans
$1/2$ cup chopped cilantro
8 whole-wheat tortillas
1 to 2 cups Cilantro Salsa (page 94)
$1 \, 1/2$ cups mozzarella-style soy cheese

1. Heat oil in large skillet. Sauté chopped onion, green peppers, mushrooms, tofu, and salt until peppers are tender and tofu is lightly browned. Stir in chili powder, cayenne, cumin, and black pepper.

2. Add beans to vegetable mixture and cook until beans are soft, adding a little water as needed. Stir in cilantro.

3. Preheat oven to 375°.

4. While beans are cooking, warm tortillas in a dry skillet. Sprinkle $1/8$ cup soy cheese on each tortilla and spoon bean mixture in the center of the tortillas. Fold in the sides of each tortilla, then roll up. Arrange burritos seam-side down in a lightly oiled casserole, cover with heated Cilantro Salsa and extra cheese, and bake for 10 minutes at 375°, or until cheese is melted and bubbly. Serve hot.

Red Pepper Tempeh

Serves 4

Tired of tofu? Try this tasty variation on soy. Tempeh combines with the slightly sweet, smoky flavor of roasted red peppers and fresh green peas for a rich but healthy dinner. Serve with brown rice and a bitter greens salad.

3 medium red peppers
1 tablespoon olive oil
$1/_2$ cup sliced button mushrooms
$1/_2$ cup chopped leeks
1 teaspoon sea salt
$1/_2$ teaspoon white pepper
1 package soybean tempeh
1 cup fresh or frozen green peas
1 tablespoon honey
$1/_2$ cup finely chopped fresh basil

1. Place peppers on a baking sheet in a 400° oven for 30 minutes, turning several times until evenly charred on all sides. Wrap peppers in a damp towel to cool, then cut in half and remove stems and seeds. Let cool.

2. While peppers are roasting, heat oil in medium skillet. Add mushrooms, leeks, salt, and pepper, and sauté over medium heat until mushrooms are limp.

3. Cut tempeh into $1/_4$-inch strips and add to skillet with vegetables. Stir in peas and cook until tempeh is lightly browned and peas are tender.

4. Slice cooled red peppers into long strips and stir into tempeh mixture. Add honey and basil, and cook just until heated through and basil wilts.

Garlic–Toasted Nut Mix

Makes 2 cups

A salty-sweet, healthy alternative to chips and other munchies. Serve as a party appetizer, or sprinkle on salads for a crunchy taste treat.

6 cloves garlic
1 tablespoon olive oil
1 tablespoon tamari
2 tablespoons honey
1 cup soybeans, soaked overnight
$^1\!/_2$ cup pepitas
$^1\!/_2$ cup walnuts or pecans

1. Peel garlic cloves and squeeze through garlic press (to make peeling cloves easier, drop into boiling water for 30 seconds—skins will slip off easily).
2. Preheat oven to 375°.
3. Heat oil in medium skillet. Sauté garlic until golden. Stir in tamari and honey.
4. Drain soybeans and add to skillet. Stir well to coat.
5. Add pepitas and walnuts or pecans, mixing well. Spread evenly on baking sheet and bake at 375° for 20 minutes, or until golden. Cool thoroughly.

Tempeh with Garlic Sauce
Serves 4

The pungent flavor of garlic with delicate snow peas adds a special twist to tempeh.
Serve over brown rice with lightly steamed greens.

1 tablespoon safflower oil
1 medium red onion, sliced
1 cup diagonally sliced carrots
1 tablespoon tamari
1 package soy tempeh, crumbled
1 cup snow peas, with stems removed
3 cloves garlic
1 tablespoon light sesame oil
1 tablespoon whole-wheat flour
$1/2$ cup vegetable stock
$1/2$ cup soy milk
$1/4$ teaspoon white pepper

1. Heat oil in large saucepan. Sauté onion, carrots, and tamari until carrots are tender.
2. Add tempeh and snow peas, and cook until tempeh is lightly browned.
3. Peel garlic cloves and mince (to make peeling cloves easier, drop into boiling water for 30 seconds—skins will slip off easily).
4. In a medium saucepan, heat sesame oil and sauté garlic until soft but not browned.
5. Add flour and stir to coat garlic. Cook for 2 to 3 minutes, stirring frequently, then slowly stir in stock, soy milk, and white pepper, cooking over low heat for 5 minutes longer, or until sauce is thick and flavors are well blended. Stir sauce into tempeh mixture and serve over rice.

Cilantro–Walnut Tofu

Serves 4

Who'd have thought plain old tofu could taste so festive? Teamed with a palate-pleasing twist on traditional pesto, this dish will make converts out of tofu haters.

$1/2$ cup walnuts
1 large bunch cilantro, coarsely chopped
3 tablespoons olive oil
3 cloves garlic, minced
1 teaspoon sea salt
$1/4$ teaspoon black pepper
1 tablespoon safflower oil
1 pound extra-firm tofu, cubed
1 head radicchio, separated into individual leaves
2 heads Belgian endive, separated into individual leaves

1. Toast walnuts at 375° for 8 to 10 minutes. Cool slightly and chop finely.
2. Combine cilantro, olive oil, walnuts, garlic, salt, and pepper in blender. Purée until very smooth, adding water as needed to make a thick sauce.
3. Heat safflower oil in a medium saucepan. Sauté tofu until lightly browned.
4. Carefully stir pesto into tofu and heat through. Arrange radicchio and endive leaves on a platter and spoon tofu-pesto mixture on top.

Super Berry Smoothie

Serves 2 to 4

No more excuses for missing a healthy breakfast. This quick and easy, low-fat shake is ideal for anyone on the go. And it makes a great cooling mid-day snack.

1 cup vanilla soy milk
$1/2$ cup apple juice
1 cup blueberries, blackberries, raspberries, or sliced strawberries
1 ripe banana
1 cup crushed ice

Combine all ingredients in blender and purée till smooth. Serve garnished with berries or slices of banana.

Spicy Tofu Steaks
Serves 6

This tangy tofu dish is ideal to prepare ahead of time. Marinate overnight, then just heat and serve with a side of lightly steamed greens for a fast, healthy meal.

1 8-ounce can tomato paste
$^1/_4$ cup tomato juice
$^1/_2$ to 1 teaspoon cayenne pepper
1 teaspoon sea salt
$^1/_2$ teaspoon black pepper
1 tablespoon honey
$^1/_4$ cup tamari
2 tablespoons finely chopped jalapeno peppers
1 pound extra-firm tofu
1 tablespoon safflower oil
1 tablespoon arrowroot
$^1/_2$ cup water
$^1/_4$ cup thinly sliced scallions (with green tops)

1. Combine tomato paste and tomato juice in a medium bowl. Add cayenne pepper, sea salt, black pepper, honey, tamari, and jalapeno peppers, and mix well.

2. Slice tofu into cutlets, about $^1/_4$-inch thick, and layer in glass casserole, lightly coated with safflower oil.

3. Pour half of marinade over tofu slices, making sure all cutlets are coated, and let marinate overnight in refrigerator.

4. To cook cutlets: lightly cover with foil and bake at 375° until warmed through and sauce is bubbly (about 10 minutes).

5. While cutlets are cooking, pour remaining marinade into small saucepan. Dissolve arrowroot into water, stir into marinade, and cook over low heat until thickened.

6. To serve, place cutlets on large platter and drizzle with hot marinade. Garnish with scallions.

Tempeh with Pine Nuts and Morels

Serves 4 to 6

Pine nuts, wild mushrooms, and crisp, green snow peas give this tempeh dish an exotic flavor. Serve with hot Walnut-Oat Bread (page 123) and a side of steamed greens for a delicious dinner treat.

$^1/_4$ cup pine nuts
1 tablespoon olive oil
1 cup sliced morel mushrooms (or other mushrooms)
$^1/_2$ cup minced shallots
1 teaspoon sea salt
$^1/_2$ teaspoon black pepper
1 package finely crumbled soy tempeh
$^1/_4$ cup chopped parsley
$^1/_4$ cup finely chopped red pepper
$^1/_4$ cup red wine
1 cup snow peas, with stems removed

1. Toast pine nuts at 375° for about 5 minutes.
2. Heat oil in medium saucepan and add mushrooms, shallots, salt, and pepper. Sauté until shallots are translucent.
3. Stir in tempeh and cook until tempeh is lightly browned and crunchy.
4. Add pine nuts, parsley, chopped red pepper, and red wine. Heat through just until red pepper is tender. Add snow peas and cook just until heated through. Serve over basmati rice.

Thelma's Raspberry Sort-Of Cheesecake
Serves 8

For a cool and refreshing, healthy summer dessert, try this low-fat version of the traditional cheesecake. It's virtually guilt free.

4 8-ounce blocks low-fat firm tofu
$1/4$ cup low-fat vanilla soy milk
1 cup Sucanat
2 teaspoons natural vanilla
2 tablespoons lemon juice
2 tablespoons arrowroot
1 deep-dish graham pie crust
$3/4$ cup raspberry preserves
Edible flowers for garnish

1. Preheat oven to 350°.
2. Purée tofu until smooth, adding soy milk as needed.
3. Combine tofu mixture with Sucanat, vanilla, and lemon juice, blending well. Stir in arrowroot dissolved in a little water.
4. Pour into crust and bake for 30 minutes at 350° until firm. Refrigerate for 30 minutes, spread raspberry preserves on top, and garnish with flowers.

11

GRAINS

**PHYTOCHEMICALS
IN WHOLE GRAINS**

phenolic acid

phytic acid

vitamin E

fiber (including lignins)

Sesame Soba Salad

Serves 4 to 6

This cold salad uses traditional Japanese buckwheat noodles with fresh vegetables, crisp water chestnuts, a sweet, nutty dressing, and lots of basil—a refreshing change of pace from tossed green salads.

1 pound dry soba noodles
1 tablespoon light sesame oil
1 cup cubed firm tofu
$1/2$ cup sliced scallions (slice and reserve green tops for garnish)
$1/2$ cup diced red pepper
2 tablespoons freshly grated ginger
$1/4$ teaspoon white pepper
1 teaspoon sea salt
$1/4$ cup coarsely chopped basil
$1/2$ cup snow peas, with stems removed
$1/2$ cup sliced water chestnuts, drained and rinsed well
$1/2$ cup tahini
$1/4$ cup rice vinegar
2 tablespoons honey
2 tablespoons white sesame seeds
2 tablespoons black sesame seeds for garnish (optional)

1. Cook soba noodles in a large soup pot with 2 quarts of water for 5 to 7 minutes, or until just tender. Drain and rinse with cold water until completely cooled.

2. While noodles are cooking, heat oil in a medium skillet and sauté tofu, scallions, red pepper, ginger, white pepper, and salt. Add basil, snow peas, and water chestnuts, and cook just until basil is wilted.

3. Combine tahini, vinegar, honey, and white sesame seeds in small bowl. Mix well.

4. In a medium mixing bowl, combine cooked noodles, vegetables, and tahini sauce and stir well to completely coat noodles. Chill thoroughly to allow flavors to combine. Garnish with black sesame seeds and green scallion tops.

Coconut-Curried Udon

Serves 4 to 6

Hot and spicy, this fragrant dish combines Japanese whole-wheat noodles with curry, coconut milk, and crunchy green celery. Serve with Sweet and Spicy Carrot Salad (page 153) on a bed of greens.

1 pound udon noodles
$^1/_4$ cup olive oil
1 small yellow onion, minced
$^1/_2$ cup finely sliced celery
$^1/_2$ cup fresh, chopped basil
1 teaspoon white pepper
1 teaspoon sea salt
2 tablespoons curry blend
1 cup light coconut milk
2 teaspoons arrowroot

1. Cook udon noodles in a large soup pot with 2 quarts of water for about 7 minutes, or until still slightly firm. Drain and set aside.

2. While noodles are cooking, heat oil in medium skillet and sauté onion, celery, basil, white pepper, and salt until onions are translucent.

3. In a small mixing bowl, combine curry blend, coconut milk, and arrowroot and stir well to mix.

4. Slowly add coconut mixture to onions and cook over low heat until mixture begins to thicken.

5. Stir in udon noodles and heat through on low heat until flavors are blended and udon is completely cooked. (Be careful not to overcook—high heat destroys the delicate taste of the coconut milk.)

Seven-Vegetable Pasta with Tarragon Glaze

Serves 4 to 6

Lots of fresh vegetables and fast-cooking pasta combine with a luscious ginger glaze for a wholesome grain dish that can be served either hot or cold.

1 pound whole-wheat pasta (rotini, elbow macaroni, shells)
2 tablespoons olive oil
$1/2$ cup sliced red onion
$1/2$ cup sliced button mushrooms
$1/2$ cup diagonally sliced carrots
$1/2$ cup broccoli florets
$1/2$ cup diced red pepper
$1/2$ cup chopped black olives
$1/2$ cup fresh green peas
1 teaspoon sea salt
2 cloves garlic, minced
$1/2$ cup finely chopped fresh tarragon (reserve a few sprigs for garnish)
2 tablespoons honey
$1/4$ teaspoon white pepper
1 tablespoon arrowroot
$1/2$ cup white wine or water

1. Cook pasta in a large soup pot with 2 quarts of water for 7 to 10 minutes, or until just tender. Rinse, drain, and set aside.

2. While pasta is cooking, heat olive oil in a large skillet and sauté onion, mushrooms, carrots, broccoli, red pepper, olives, peas, and salt until carrots and broccoli are tender.

3. In a small saucepan, sauté garlic, tarragon, honey, and white pepper. Dissolve arrowroot in wine or water, slowly stir into tarragon mixture, and cook until thick and bubbly.

4. Add tarragon glaze to cooked vegetables. Combine in a large serving bowl with pasta and serve hot.

Wild Rice Salad with Toasted Pecans
Serves 4

Wild rice, crunchy toasted pecans, and fresh green peas combine in this nutty start to any meal. Or serve it hot as a side dish with broiled fish and steamed greens.

$^1/_4$ cup chopped pecans
1 tablespoon olive oil
$^1/_2$ cup sliced shiitake mushrooms or button mushrooms
1 large leek, thinly sliced (with green top)
1 teaspoon sea salt
$^1/_2$ cup grated carrot
$^1/_2$ cup fresh or frozen green peas
1 cup cooked wild rice
1 cup cooked brown rice
$^1/_4$ teaspoon white pepper
$^1/_2$ teaspoon black pepper

1. Toast pecans at 375° for 8 to 10 minutes.
2. While pecans are toasting, heat oil in medium saucepan and sauté shiitakes, sliced leek, and salt until leek slices begin to turn translucent. Stir in grated carrot and peas and cook until peas are just tender (about 5 minutes).
3. Combine wild rice, brown rice, pecans, white pepper, and black pepper in medium mixing bowl.
4. Add shiitake mixture to rice mixture, blend well, and chill thoroughly. Serve on a bed of lightly steamed bitter greens, or serve hot as a side dish.

Millet and Summer Squash Casserole

Serves 6 to 8

A satisfying, creamy meal-in-a-dish that combines the unique taste of often overlooked millet with delicately sweet summer squash.

2 cups cooked millet
1 ½ cups grated mozzarella-style soy cheese
½ cup silken tofu, blended
½ cup chopped fresh basil
1 teaspoon sea salt
½ teaspoon black pepper
1 tablespoon olive oil
2 cups sliced summer squash
1 medium green pepper, sliced into thin rings
1 medium red onion, thinly sliced

1. Preheat oven to 350°.

2. Combine millet, 1 cup of the soy cheese, tofu, basil, salt, and pepper in a medium saucepan. Heat until cheese melts and custard becomes thick and creamy.

3. Coat the bottom of a glass casserole with oil and spoon in half of millet mixture. Arrange squash, green pepper, and onion on top, and spread remaining millet mixture on top of vegetables.

4. Sprinkle remaining soy cheese on top of casserole and bake at 350° for 20 minutes. Let cool slightly to set before serving.

Spicy Pepper Pasta
Serves 4 to 6

A hot and spicy take on plain old spaghetti. Serve as a rich dinner meal with a cold salad of mixed greens and fresh vegetables, and hot garlic bread.

1 pound whole-wheat spaghetti
1 tablespoon olive oil
2 cloves garlic, minced
$\frac{1}{2}$ cup sliced red onion
$\frac{1}{2}$ cup chopped celery
$\frac{1}{2}$ cup hot green peppers
$\frac{1}{2}$ cup sliced button mushrooms
1 teaspoon sea salt
1 teaspoon black pepper
$\frac{1}{2}$ teaspoon cayenne pepper
$\frac{1}{2}$ cup diced tomatoes
$\frac{1}{2}$ cup finely chopped fresh oregano
$\frac{1}{2}$ cup red wine
$\frac{1}{2}$ to 1 teaspoon hot red pepper flakes

1. Cook spaghetti in a large soup pot with 2 quarts of water for 8 to 10 minutes, or until just tender.

2. While pasta is cooking, heat olive oil in a large skillet and sauté garlic, onion, celery, hot green peppers, mushrooms, salt, black pepper, and cayenne pepper until vegetables are tender. Stir in tomatoes and oregano, and cook for 3 to 5 minutes longer, until tomatoes are soft.

3. Stir in red wine and red pepper flakes. Rinse and drain pasta, add to vegetable mixture, and stir until well coated.

Cilantro–Walnut Tabouli

Serves 4

Try this tasty variation on the traditional Middle Eastern favorite. It's a quick, easy way to add nutritious whole grains to any meal.

1 cup dry cracked wheat bulgur
2 cups hot water
$1/4$ cup finely chopped walnuts
$1/2$ cup finely chopped cilantro
$1/4$ cup finely chopped parsley
1 tablespoon vinegar
2 tablespoons olive oil
2 cloves garlic, minced
1 teaspoon sea salt
1 teaspoon white pepper

1. Soak bulgur overnight in water, or combine water and bulgur in a medium saucepan, bring to a boil, remove from heat, and let stand, covered, until bulgur is soft. Drain excess liquid.

2. Toast walnuts in a 375° oven for 5 to 8 minutes.

3. Combine cilantro and parsley in a medium bowl. Stir in vinegar, olive oil, garlic, sea salt, pepper, and toasted walnuts.

4. Add cooked or soaked bulgur to cilantro mixture and mix well. Chill well to allow flavors to blend.

Fragrant Spiced Basmati Rice
Serves 4 to 6

Nutty-tasting, whole-grain basmati rice combines with cardamom, saffron, and fresh green peas to make an exotic, delicately spiced side dish for fish or tempeh dishes. It's also a great lunch treat all on its own.

4 cups water
1 teaspoon sea salt
2 cups whole-grain basmati rice
1 tablespoon olive oil
2 cloves garlic, minced
1 teaspoon ground cardamom
$^1/_2$ teaspoon ground saffron
1 teaspoon cumin seed
$^1/_4$ teaspoon white pepper
$^1/_4$ cup fresh green peas, shelled
$^1/_4$ cup pine nuts (optional)

1. Bring water and salt to boil and stir in basmati rice. Lower heat and cook, covered, for 30 to 45 minutes, or until rice is tender.

2. While rice is cooking, heat oil in a small skillet and sauté garlic, cardamom, saffron, cumin seed, and white pepper. Stir in peas and cook until tender.

3. Stir spice mixture into cooked rice. Add pine nuts if desired.

Walnut–Oat Bread

Makes one loaf

A healthy, hearty nut- and grain-packed quick bread to serve with almost any meal. Fresh and hot from the oven, it's a mouth-watering treat all by itself.

1 cup coarsely chopped walnuts
2 cups whole-wheat flour
$1/2$ cup oats
$1/2$ teaspoon baking soda
1 teaspoon aluminum-free baking powder
1 teaspoon salt
1 $1/2$ cups soy milk
$1/2$ cup silken tofu
$1/4$ cup honey
2 tablespoons safflower oil

1. Toast walnuts at 375° for 8 to 10 minutes.
2. Combine flour, oats, baking soda, baking powder, and salt in a medium bowl. Mix well to combine.
3. Puree soy milk, tofu, and honey in a blender until very smooth. Stir tofu mixture into flour and blend well. Stir in toasted walnuts.
4. Coat loaf pan with oil and turn batter into pan. Bake at 350° for 45 minutes to 1 hour, or until completely cooked in the center (until a toothpick comes out clean).
5. Cool for 20 to 30 minutes, turn out of pan, and serve.

Whole-Wheat Fettuccini with Salmon and Sage
Serves 4 to 6

Savory sage and hearty salmon combine with whole-grain pasta for a delicious dinner treat. This versatile dish also makes a great cold salad for leftover lunches.

1 pound fresh salmon fillet
1 pound whole-wheat fettuccini
1 teaspoon salt
1 tablespoon olive oil
$^1/_2$ cup sliced yellow onion
$^1/_2$ cup sliced mushrooms (morel, button, shiitake, or other)
2 cloves garlic, minced
$^1/_4$ cup chopped fresh sage
$^1/_4$ cup red wine

1. Wash salmon thoroughly, remove skin and bones, and cut into 1-inch chunks.

2. Cook fettuccini with salt in a large soup pot with 2 quarts of water for 7 to 10 minutes, or until just tender.

3. While pasta is cooking, heat oil in a medium skillet and sauté sliced onion, mushrooms, and garlic over medium heat just until onion begins to turn translucent.

4. Stir in sage and increase heat until sage begins to brown. Lower heat, and add red wine and salmon. Cover and simmer until salmon is thoroughly cooked.

5. Drain pasta, arrange on a serving platter, and lightly toss with salmon-sage mixture.

12

CITRUS FRUITS

**PHYTOCHEMICALS
IN CITRUS FRUITS**

vitamin C

terpenes (including limonoids)

glutathione

Citrus Salad with Spiced Raisins and Jicama
Serves 4

Raisins spiked with clove, nutmeg, and cinnamon add a sweet and zesty flavor to this tangy, refreshing combination of citrus fruits, exotic jicama, and crunchy pecans. Nice for a light summer salad, dessert, or special breakfast treat.

$1/2$ cup chopped pecans
$1/2$ cup raisins
$1/2$ cup warm water
1 tablespoon ground cinnamon
1 tablespoon ground cloves
1 tablespoon ground nutmeg
2 tablespoons honey
1 small grapefruit
2 medium oranges
2 medium tangerines
$1/2$ cup peeled and cubed jicama

1. Toast pecans at 375° for 5 to 8 minutes.

2. In a medium saucepan, combine raisins, water, cinnamon, cloves, nutmeg, and honey. Bring to a boil, then reduce heat and let simmer until all water is absorbed. Let cool.

3. Cut grapefruit in half and spoon out sections. Place in medium mixing bowl. Peel oranges and tangerines, divide into sections, and combine with grapefruit.

4. Stir raisins into fruit mixture. Add jicama and toasted pecans. Chill thoroughly before serving.

Iced Berry Lemonade
Serves 4 to 6

A refreshing summer drink that combines tart lemons with sweet raspberries and blueberries. Serve in tall, frosted glasses, garnished with sprigs of mint.

$^1/_2$ cup fresh-squeezed lemon juice
$^1/_4$ cup honey
2 tea bags
$^1/_2$ cup blueberries
$^1/_2$ cup raspberries
3 cups water

1. Combine lemon juice and honey in small saucepan. Heat on low just until honey is melted. Add tea bags and let steep for 3 to 5 minutes.

2. Purée lemon-honey mixture with blueberries, raspberries, and water until very smooth. Chill thoroughly.

3. Rinse four tall glasses with cold water and place in freezer for 5 minutes, or until frosted. Add crushed ice and serve Iced Berry Lemonade in frosted glasses, garnished with sprigs of mint or additional berries.

Grapefruit and Kiwi Salad on Field Greens
Serves 4

Tangy grapefruit, sweet kiwi, and juicy blackberries make a marvelous medley in this colorful summer salad.

$^1/_4$ cup raspberry vinegar
2 tablespoons olive oil
1 tablespoon honey
1 cup grapefruit sections
1 cup peeled and sliced kiwi
1 cup fresh blackberries
2 cups mixed field greens

1. In a small mixing bowl, combine vinegar, oil, and honey, mixing until well blended.

2. Combine grapefruit, kiwi, and blackberries in medium bowl. Add vinaigrette and stir gently to coat fruit well.

3. Arrange field greens on serving platter and spoon fruit mixture on top. Chill before serving.

Asparagus with Ginger–Orange Glaze
Serves 4 to 6

Hot or cold, this refreshing dish is a luscious, fat-free combination of asparagus and tart citrus fruits, with a hint of cumin and spicy ginger.

1 pound asparagus
$^1/_4$ cup fresh grated ginger
$^3/_4$ cup freshly squeezed orange juice
2 tablespoons lemon juice
1 teaspoon honey
1 teaspoon ground cumin
$^1/_2$ teaspoon white pepper
$^1/_2$ teaspoon sea salt
1 tablespoon arrowroot

1. Wash asparagus well, break off tough ends, and steam until tender (about 10 minutes).

2. While asparagus is steaming, combine ginger, orange juice, lemon juice, honey, cumin, pepper, and salt in small saucepan. Bring to a near boil.

3. Dissolve arrowroot in a small amount of water and slowly add to orange juice mixture. Lower heat and let mixture cook over low, stirring frequently, until thick and glossy.

4. Arrange asparagus on serving platter and drizzle glaze over top. To serve cold, rinse asparagus under very cold water after steaming and toss with glaze. Refrigerate until well chilled.

Dreamy Orange-Cream Freeze
Serves 4

This creamy, dreamy dessert or anytime snack is deliciously low in fat and completely dairy free. A super-fast, guilt-free treat for any occasion.

2 cups freshly squeezed orange juice
$^1/_2$ cup low-fat soy yogurt
$^1/_2$ cup low-fat soy milk
Orange slices for garnish

1. Combine orange juice, soy yogurt, and soy milk in a blender. Purée until thick and creamy.
2. Freeze juice mixture for 1 hour, stirring every 15 minutes until smooth.
3. Let warm slightly and spoon into individual serving dishes. Garnish with orange slices.

Honeydew Lime Cooler
Serves 4

The flavors of sweet honeydew, tart lime, and juicy red grapes combine in this smooth summer drink. A refreshing change of pace from sodas and iced tea.

1 small honeydew melon
$^1/_2$ cup seedless red grapes
$^1/_2$ cup freshly squeezed lime juice
$^1/_2$ cup honey
2 cups sparkling water

1. Cut melon in half, scoop out seeds, peel, and cut into 1-inch cubes. Wash grapes well and remove stems. Freeze melon and grapes for one hour.
2. Combine frozen melon and grapes with lime juice and honey in a blender. Purée until smooth, adding water as needed. Serve immediately.

Skinny Lemon Caper Sauce
Makes 2 cups

This creamy, special sauce is low-fat and dairy-free, with the distinctive flavors of capers, tangy lemon, pungent garlic, and a whisper of spicy ginger. So rich and flavorful, you'll swear it's decadent.

2 tablespoons olive oil
3 garlic cloves, minced
$1/2$ teaspoon white pepper
$1/2$ teaspoon sea salt
2 teaspoons finely grated fresh ginger
1 tablespoon whole-wheat flour
$1/2$ cup vegetable stock
$1/2$ cup soy milk
$1/2$ cup lemon juice
$1/4$ cup capers

1. In a medium saucepan, heat oil and sauté garlic, pepper, salt, and ginger until garlic is golden.

2. Add flour and stir to coat garlic and ginger. Cook for 2 to 3 minutes, stirring frequently. Slowly stir in stock and soy milk. Simmer for 3 to 5 minutes longer, stirring frequently, until sauce is thick and creamy.

3. Place lemon juice in small mixing bowl. Carefully whisk in hot soy milk mixture a little at a time. Beat vigorously until creamy and smooth.

4. Return to pan, add capers, and heat through on very low heat. Serve immediately as a glaze over broiled fish or sauce for hot vegetables.

Blood Orange Ambrosia

Serves 4 to 6

With its combination of blood oranges, coconut, pecans, and sweet, juicy fruits, this low-fat dessert lives up to its name—truly ambrosial.

$^1/_2$ cup chopped pecans
1 cup blood orange sections (tangerines or navel oranges may be
      substituted)
1 banana, sliced on the diagonal
$^1/_2$ cup blackberries
1 very ripe peach, sliced
$^1/_2$ cup seedless red grapes
1 cup low-fat soy yogurt
1 teaspoon vanilla
2 tablespoons honey
$^1/_2$ cup coconut

1. Toast pecans at 375° for 5 to 8 minutes.
2. Combine orange sections, banana slices, blackberries, peach slices, and grapes in medium mixing bowl.
3. In small bowl, combine soy yogurt, vanilla, and honey, and mix well. Stir in coconut and toasted pecans.
4. Toss fruit with soy-yogurt dressing and chill before serving.

Tangerine Dream
Serves 4

Presentation is everything in this simple summer salad. The unique taste of tangerines pairs up with blueberries and extra-ripe pears, artfully arranged on a bed of Bibb lettuce and garnished with fruit glaze and edible flowers.

$^1/_2$ cup tangerine juice (orange juice may be substituted)
1 tablespoon arrowroot
2 tablespoons honey
1 small head Bibb or oak-leaf lettuce
3 to 4 tangerines, peeled and separated into sections
1 cup blueberries
2 ripe pears, peeled, cored, and cut into eighths
Edible flowers for garnish (optional)

1. Combine tangerine juice, arrowroot, and honey in a small saucepan. Bring to a boil, stirring constantly, then remove immediately from heat. Refrigerate to cool thoroughly.

2. While sauce is cooling, core lettuce, gently separate leaves, and immerse completely in ice-cold water to remove all sand and dirt. Drain, rinse well, and pat dry. Place on decorative individual serving dishes.

3. Arrange pear slices in a circle on top of lettuce on each dish. Arrange tangerine sections in a smaller circle. Place $^1/_4$ cup of blueberries in the center of pear and tangerine circle on each dish.

4. Drizzle chilled glaze lightly over each fruit plate and garnish with edible flowers, if desired. Serve immediately.

Lemonberry Muffins
Makes 12 muffins

The tart taste of lemon is a perfect complement to the blueberries in these tender little muffins. Low in fat and high in nutrition, they're a great way to start your day or end your dinner.

1 cup unbleached white flour
2 cups whole-wheat flour
1 tablespoon baking powder
1 teaspoon sea salt
$\frac{1}{2}$ cup honey
1 cup soy milk
$\frac{1}{4}$ cup safflower oil
$\frac{1}{2}$ cup lemon juice
1 cup blueberries

1. Preheat oven to 375°.
2. Combine unbleached white and whole-wheat flours with baking powder and sea salt. Mix well.
3. In a separate bowl, mix honey, soy milk, and safflower oil. Beat in lemon juice until smooth.
4. Add soy-milk mixture to flour mixture and blend just until all ingredients are combined. Gently fold in blueberries.
5. Pour batter into muffin tins lined with paper muffin cups. Bake at 375° for 20 minutes, or until cooked completely in center (test with a toothpick). Let cool before serving.

13

GREENS

**PHYTOCHEMICALS
IN GREENS**

vitamin C

vitamin A

folic acid

carotenoids (including lutein

and beta-carotene)

Curried Greens

Serves 4 to 6

Eating your greens comes easy when they're served up spicy with this pungent, fragrant sauce. Serve with broiled fish and steamed whole-grain basmati rice.

2 tablespoons olive oil
1 medium yellow onion, diced
2 cloves garlic, minced
1 cup diced red potatoes
1 cup vegetable stock
1 tablespoon dried curry blend
1 teaspoon sea salt
1 teaspoon black pepper
1 tablespoon arrowroot, dissolved in a little water
$^{1}/_{2}$ pound turnip greens, coarsely chopped
$^{1}/_{2}$ pound kale, coarsely chopped

1. Heat oil in large soup pan. Sauté onion and garlic until onion is translucent. Add potatoes and stock, cover, and simmer until potatoes are tender (about 7 minutes).

2. Stir in curry, salt, and pepper, mixing well. Add arrowroot and simmer until sauce begins to thicken.

3. Add turnip greens and kale, and cook until greens are bright green and tender.

Creamy Spinach Sage Soup
Serves 4 to 6

This dairy-free delight, with delicate undertones of sage, is a wonderful way to serve up spinach. Low in fat and loaded with calcium, it's a super-healthy soup in disguise.

1 tablespoon olive oil
1 medium leek, sliced (without green tops)
1 teaspoon sea salt
$1/4$ teaspoon white pepper
2 tablespoons fresh sage, finely chopped (reserve a few sprigs for garnish)
2 tablespoons whole-wheat flour
4 cups vegetable stock
1 pound spinach, torn into large pieces, with stems removed
1 8-ounce container silken low-fat tofu, cubed
Red pepper and sage for garnish

1. In large soup pot, heat olive oil and sauté sliced leek with salt until slices are soft.

2. Add white pepper, sage, and flour, and cook for 2 to 3 minutes, stirring constantly.

3. Slowly stir in vegetable stock. Add spinach and cook until spinach is soft.

4. Purée mixture with tofu until well-blended and creamy. Return to pan and heat through. Garnish with thin slices of red pepper and additional sprigs of fresh sage.

Spinach–Mushroom Samosas

Serves 10

These tasty, traditional Indian pastries are baked instead of fried for a substantial savings in fat and calories. Serve them as appetizers or spicy side dishes.

Dough:
2 cups whole-wheat flour
1 teaspoon salt
2 tablespoons safflower oil
$^3/_4$ cup water

Filling:
1 tablespoon safflower oil
$^1/_2$ cup chopped onion
1 cup sliced button mushrooms
1 tablespoon cumin seeds
1 teaspoon ground coriander
1 teaspoon turmeric
1 tablespoon freshly ground ginger
$^1/_2$ teaspoon black pepper
1 teaspoon sea salt
1 cup firm tofu, mashed
1 pound spinach, torn into small pieces with stems removed
6 medium red potatoes, peeled, boiled, and mashed

1. To make dough, mix flour, salt, and oil, adding water gradually as needed to form a stiff dough. Cover and let rest for about 20 minutes.

2. In a medium skillet, heat oil and sauté chopped onion and mushrooms until golden. Add cumin seeds, coriander, turmeric, ginger, pepper, and salt. Cook for about 1 minute.

3. Stir in tofu and sauté for about 5 minutes. Add spinach and cook just until spinach turns bright green and begins to wilt. Remove from heat and let cool.

4. In a medium mixing bowl, combine cooled spinach and tofu mixture with mashed potatoes. Mix well.

5. Preheat oven to 375°.

6. Divide dough into 10 balls and roll into thin circles about 4 inches in diameter, adding flour as needed. Spoon filling into center of each circle of dough. Moisten dough edge with water and fold circle in half, pinching edges together firmly with fingers or fork to seal.

7. Lightly coat a cookie sheet with oil and arrange samosas on the sheet so they're not touching. Bake at 375° for 30 to 40 minutes, or until golden brown. Serve hot.

Collard and Carrot Raita
Serves 6 to 8

This yogurt-based salad is traditionally served as a cooling accompaniment to hot and spicy Indian dishes. Try it with Indian Vegetable Curry (page 97).

$\frac{1}{2}$ pound collard greens, chopped
2 cups soy yogurt
$\frac{1}{2}$ cup shredded carrot
$\frac{1}{4}$ cup raisins
1 teaspoon sea salt
$\frac{1}{2}$ teaspoon black pepper
1 teaspoon ground cumin

1. Lightly steam collard greens, just until bright green. Rinse under cold water to stop cooking.
2. Blend yogurt with carrot, raisins, salt, pepper, and cumin.
3. Stir in cooled collard greens. Chill thoroughly before serving.

Braised Swiss Chard
Serves 4 to 6

Radicchio and currants combine with fresh green Swiss chard for an appealing side dish. Serve with fish dishes, or over brown rice for a light lunch.

1 tablespoon olive oil
2 medium shallots, minced
$\frac{1}{2}$ cup water
1 pound Swiss chard, torn into large pieces with stems removed
1 teaspoon sea salt
1 teaspoon white pepper
$\frac{1}{2}$ cup currants
1 medium head of radicchio, cored and cut into 12 wedges

1. Heat oil in medium skillet and sauté shallots until soft.
2. Stir in water, Swiss chard, salt, pepper, and currants, and cook until chard is bright green.
3. Add radicchio and cook over medium heat just until radicchio wilts. Serve hot.

Palak Paneer

Serves 4 to 6

Try this dairy-free take on a traditional Indian favorite. Served with hot pita bread as an appetizer, it's sure to please anyone who otherwise doesn't eat greens.

1 tablespoon safflower oil
1 cup firm tofu, cubed
1 medium yellow onion, diced
1 teaspoon ground cumin
1 teaspoon coriander
$1/2$ teaspoon turmeric
1 teaspoon sea salt
$1/2$ teaspoon white pepper
$1/2$ cup soy milk
$3/4$ pound spinach, torn into medium pieces with stems removed

1. Heat oil in medium skillet and sauté tofu and diced onion until tofu begins to turn golden. Add cumin, coriander, turmeric, salt, and pepper.

2. Briefly puree soy milk and spinach.

3. Add spinach mixture to tofu mixture in skillet and cook over low heat for 15 minutes. Serve warm.

Southern Style Turnip Greens

Serves 4

Try this low-fat take on the traditional, down-South version of turnip greens—all the taste, minus the pork and hours of boiling.

1 tablespoon safflower oil
1 small yellow onion, minced
1 teaspoon sea salt
$1/2$ teaspoon black pepper
$1/2$ cup water
2 cups diced turnips
1 pound turnip greens, torn into medium-sized pieces, with stems removed
2 tablespoons red wine vinegar

1. Heat oil in a medium skillet and sauté minced onion, salt, and pepper until onion is translucent.

2. Add water and turnips, cover, and cook just until turnips are tender.

3. Add turnip greens and steam until greens are tender and turnips are soft. Stir in vinegar and serve hot.

Mixed Greens Stew

Serves 4 to 6

A delicious medley of mixed greens combines with garbanzo beans and lots of garlic in this hearty dish. Serve with sourdough bread as a meal in itself.

1 tablespoon olive oil
2 bunches scallions, thinly sliced
4 cloves garlic, minced
1 tablespoon whole-wheat flour
4 cups vegetable stock
$\frac{1}{2}$ teaspoon sea salt
1 teaspoon white pepper
1 $\frac{1}{2}$ cups cooked garbanzo beans
1 cup beet greens, chopped
1 cup kale, chopped
1 cup spinach, chopped
1 cup chard, chopped

1. In a large soup pot, heat oil and sauté scallions and garlic until scallions are soft.

2. Stir in flour and cook for 2 to 3 minutes. Slowly add stock, salt, and pepper, and cook until slightly thickened.

3. Add beans and greens, and simmer for 10 to 15 minutes, or until greens are tender.

Baked Kale with Parsnips and Carrots
Serves 6 to 8

This fast, healthy casserole pairs parsnips and carrots with tangy kale and red wine. A quick and easy way to make sure you're getting your greens.

1 tablespoon olive oil
1 medium red onion, diced
1 $^1/_2$ cups diagonally sliced carrots
1 $^1/_2$ cups diagonally sliced parsnips
$^1/_2$ teaspoon black pepper
3 cups fresh kale, chopped, with stems removed
$^1/_4$ cup water
2 tablespoons tamari

1. Preheat oven to 350°.
2. In a medium skillet, heat oil and sauté diced onion, carrots, parsnips, and pepper until carrots and parsnips are barely tender.
3. While carrots are cooking, lightly steam kale, just until bright green (3 to 5 minutes).
4. Stir greens into carrot mixture and turn into lightly oiled glass casserole.
5. Combine water and tamari, and pour over the top of casserole. Cover loosely with foil, and bake at 350° for 15 minutes.

Spicy Gingered Greens
Serves 4 to 6

Hot or cold, this sweet and spicy dish adds an oriental flair to chard and mustard greens. Serve chilled as a salad or hot as a colorful side dish with any meal.

1 tablespoon light sesame oil
2 carrots, grated
$^1/_4$ cup freshly grated ginger
2 teaspoons tamari
2 tablespoons honey
1 tablespoon mellow white miso
1 tablespoon rice vinegar
$^1/_2$ teaspoon cayenne pepper
1 pound chard, torn into large pieces, with stems removed
1 pound mustard greens, torn into large pieces, with stems removed
$^1/_4$ cup sesame seeds
$^1/_4$ cup water

1. In a medium pan, heat oil and sauté carrots and ginger until carrots are tender.

2. While carrots are cooking, in a small bowl combine tamari, honey, miso, vinegar, and cayenne pepper, adding water as needed to form a smooth paste.

3. Add chard, mustard greens, and sesame seeds to pan with carrots, and cook just until greens are wilted.

4. Add water and miso paste to vegetables, stirring well to coat all ingredients. Serve hot, or refrigerate until completely chilled and serve cold.

14

RED/ORANGE/
YELLOW FRUITS

**PHYTOCHEMICALS
IN RED/ORANGE/YELLOW
FRUITS**

vitamin C

vitamin A

fiber

phenols (including ellagic acid)

carotenoids (including beta-carotene,

alpha-carotene, lutein, cryptoxanthin,

lycopene, zeaxanthin, canthaxanthin)

Very Berry Sauce
Makes 3 cups

This colorful concoction, with its many, mingled berry flavors, is a perfect substitute for syrup or jam on waffles, pancakes, or morning muffins.

1 cup blueberries
1 cup raspberries
$1/2$ cup sliced strawberries
$1/4$ cup rice milk
1 tablespoon arrowroot
$1/4$ cup water
$1/4$ cup honey

1. Purée blueberries, raspberries, strawberries, and rice milk until smooth.
2. Dissolve arrowroot in water and combine with berry mixture in a medium saucepan.
3. Stir in honey and bring to a slow boil. Let mixture simmer for 3 to 5 minutes, or until thick and bubbly. Refrigerate until completely chilled.

Watermelon Slushie
Serves 4

What could be easier than sweet, juicy watermelon whipped into a delicious, fat-free slush? A truly guilt-free delight.

3 cups cubed fresh watermelon
$1/2$ cup cold herbal tea
$1/2$ cup seltzer
1 small bunch fresh mint leaves

1. Freeze watermelon overnight in medium plastic container.
2. Combine frozen watermelon with herbal tea and seltzer, and purée until thick and smooth. Garnish with sprigs of fresh mint.

Veronica's Very Special Apricot Peach Tart
Serves 8 to 10

This sweet, juicy tart is lower in fat than the average dessert and loaded with lots of healthy, fresh apricots and peaches. Serve it after a very special meal.

1 ¹/₂ cups whole-wheat pastry flour
³/₄ cup whole oats
1 teaspoon sea salt
2 tablespoons safflower oil
1 cup apricot juice
2 cups sliced ripe apricots
2 cups sliced very ripe peaches
2 tablespoons whole-wheat flour
¹/₂ cup honey
¹/₄ cup sunflower oil

1. Preheat oven to 375°.
2. Combine pastry flour, ¹/₂ cup oats, and salt. Mix well.
3 Stir in oil and apricot juice, mixing until dough forms a ball. Roll out on a lightly floured surface, adding flour as needed. Press into a glass pie pan or small casserole.
4. Combine apricot and peach slices, flour, and ¹/₄ cup honey. Pour into crust.
5. Combine remaining oats and honey with sunflower oil. Mix well and sprinkle over fruit filling. Bake at 375° for 30 minutes, or until fruit is soft and juicy and topping is lightly browned.

Raspberry–Pecan Crunch

Serves 4 to 6

Fresh, juicy raspberries team up with whole grains and lots of nuts in this super-healthy dessert dish—so nutritious, you can serve it as breakfast!

$^1/_2$ cup pecans
4 cups raspberries
$^1/_4$ cup honey
$^1/_4$ cup sunflower oil
1 cup uncooked rolled oats
1 cup silken tofu
1 tablespoon vanilla
$^1/_4$ cup rice syrup

1. Toast pecans at 375° for 8 to 10 minutes. Cool slightly and chop finely.
2. Layer raspberries in lightly oiled, medium glass casserole dish.
3. Combine honey and oil, mixing until smooth.
4. Mix oats and toasted pecans, and stir in honey mixture. Sprinkle on top of raspberries. Bake at 350° for 20 minutes, or until raspberries are soft and topping is golden.
5. While raspberries are baking, purée tofu with vanilla and rice syrup until very smooth. Drizzle tofu-vanilla cream over raspberry crunch and serve hot.

Mixed Greens with Mango Glaze

Serves 4 to 6

The bitter taste of chicory and endive are complemented by super-sweet mangos and crunchy almonds in this dinner-party salad.

1 cup chicory
1 cup arugula
$^1/_2$ cup red oak leaf lettuce
1 medium head of radicchio
2 medium heads Belgian endive
2 tablespoons almond oil
$^1/_4$ cup raspberry vinegar
$^1/_2$ cup very ripe, mashed mango
1 teaspoon sea salt
$^1/_4$ teaspoon white pepper
$^1/_2$ cup sliced almonds

1. Immerse chicory, arugula, and red oak leaf lettuce completely in ice-cold water to remove all sand and dirt. Drain, rinse again, and pat dry. Tear into bite-size pieces and place in large salad bowl.

2. Rinse radicchio and endive. Core radicchio and cut into 8 wedges. Slice endive into $^1/_4$-inch slices, and add radicchio and endive to other greens. Toss well.

3. In a small mixing bowl, combine oil, vinegar, mashed mango, salt, and pepper. Mix until very smooth.

4. Add dressing to salad and mix well to coat. Sprinkle on almonds, toss again, and chill thoroughly before serving.

Red Grapefruit Ambrosia

Serves 4 to 6

For a taste of the tropics, try this sweet and tangy salad. The combination of juicy fruits and currants spiked with wine makes this dish an unusual treat.

$1/4$ cup red wine
2 tablespoons honey
$1/4$ cup currants
1 cup red grapefruit wedges
1 cup diagonally sliced bananas
1 cup cubed papaya
1 cup sliced mango
$1/2$ cup blackberries
$1/2$ cup shredded, unsweetened coconut

1. Combine red wine and honey, mixing until honey is completely dissolved. Add currants and refrigerate overnight.

2. Combine grapefruit, bananas, papaya, mango, blackberries, and $1/2$ cup coconut in a medium mixing bowl.

3. Gently stir in currants and serve in individual dishes, garnished with extra coconut.

Cantaloupe Wedges with
Frosted Champagne Grapes

Serves 4

This simple but exotic combination of fresh, sweet cantaloupe and delicately frosted champagne grapes is a wonderful, fat-free dessert to end any meal in style.

1 bunch champagne grapes
$^1/_2$ cup honey
1 teaspoon vanilla
1 medium cantaloupe
1 small bunch fresh mint leaves

1. Rinse grapes well and remove from stems. Pat dry.

2. In a small saucepan, combine honey and vanilla, and heat on low flame until honey begins to thin. Remove from heat and let cool slightly.

3. Gently stir grapes into honey mixture until well coated. Spread on a cookie sheet and freeze for half an hour.

4. While grapes are freezing, cut cantaloupe in half and remove seeds. Cut each half into 8 wedges and peel wedges. Arrange in individual dishes and chill thoroughly.

5. Remove grapes from freezer and carefully sprinkle over cantaloupe. Garnish with fresh mint and serve immediately.

Mango–Banana Freeze

Serves 4

This creamy combination of mangos and bananas makes the perfect dessert after spicy meals or a wonderful light snack for steamy summer days.

2 medium, very ripe mangos
4 ripe bananas
1 cup rice milk
$^1/_2$ cup coconut milk
1 cup crushed ice
$^1/_4$ cup unsweetened coconut flakes

1. Peel mangos and cut into chunks, scraping extra flesh off insides of skin. Peel bananas and slice.

2. Combine mangos, bananas, rice milk, coconut milk, and crushed ice in blender, and purée until thick and smooth. Stir in half of coconut flakes.

3. Freeze mixture for about 30 minutes in individual dishes. Sprinkle with remaining coconut and serve

Mango–Raisin Salsa

Makes 2 cups

Try this delicately sweet, exotic alternative to tomato salsa as a savory dipping sauce for chips or as a side for almost any fish dish.

2 medium mangos
$^1/_2$ cup raisins
1 small red onion, sliced
$^1/_2$ cup pineapple, cubed
$^1/_2$ cup honey
$^1/_2$ cup rice vinegar
$^1/_2$ cup apple juice
$^1/_2$ teaspoon cumin

1. Carefully peel and cube mangos and place in medium bowl. Scrape flesh from insides of skin and add to bowl.

2. Add raisins, onion, and pineapple to mangos and mix well.

3. Combine honey, vinegar, apple juice, and cumin in a medium saucepan. Bring to a full boil, then simmer for 15 minutes until slightly thickened.

4. Stir mango mixture into honey mixture and mix well. Chill thoroughly to allow flavors to blend and serve cold.

Strawberry Dream Pie
Serves 8

This strawberry pie is a truly dreamy dessert. Made with a pecan-spiked crust and a creamy, dairy-free filling, it's a special treat for any occasion.

2 cups crushed natural graham crackers
$1/4$ cup finely chopped pecans
$1/4$ cup safflower oil
4 cups fresh sliced strawberries
2 tablespoons lemon juice
1 cup silken tofu
$1/2$ cup rice syrup
1 teaspoon vanilla
Additional whole strawberries for garnish

1. Preheat oven to 350°.
2. Combine graham crackers, pecans, and oil. Mix well and press into a glass pie pan. Bake at 350° for 10 minutes. Remove from oven and let cool.
3. While crust is baking, combine strawberries with lemon juice. Set aside.
4. Combine tofu, rice syrup, and vanilla, and purée until very smooth. Stir in strawberries and spoon into crust.
5. Bake at 350° for another 7 minutes, or until berries are soft and juicy. Remove from oven and cool thoroughly in refrigerator to set. Garnish with additional berries and serve cold.

15

RED/ORANGE/ YELLOW VEGETABLES

PHYTOCHEMICALS IN RED/ORANGE/YELLOW VEGETABLES

vitamin C

vitamin A

fiber

phenols (including ellagic acid)

carotenoids (including beta-carotene,

alpha-carotene, lutein, cryptoxanthin,

lycopene, zeaxanthin, canthaxanthin)

Sweet and Spicy Carrot Salad
Serves 4

Try this fresh alternative to green salads—pungent spices make it a perfect start for almost any meal. Serve on a bed of field greens for an extra-special salad.

2 cups grated carrot
$^{1}/_{4}$ cup raisins
1 bunch scallions, thinly sliced, with green tops
1 cup silken tofu
1 tablespoon light sesame oil
1 teaspoon ground cumin
$^{1}/_{2}$ teaspoon nutmeg
$^{1}/_{2}$ teaspoon black pepper
1 teaspoon sea salt
2 tablespoons honey

   1. Combine grated carrot, raisins, and scallions in a medium mixing bowl.

   2. Purée tofu, sesame oil, cumin, nutmeg, pepper, salt, and honey until very smooth.

   3. Add tofu mixture to carrot mixture and blend well. Chill thoroughly to allow flavors to blend.

RED/ORANGE/
YELLOW VEGETABLES

Hearty Pumpkin Soup with Pepitas
Serves 4

Subtle spices and crunchy pepitas combine to make this creamy, dairy-free soup a delightful dish served either hot or cold.

2 tablespoons olive oil
1 small yellow onion, minced
1 teaspoon sea salt
1 teaspoon white pepper
2 tablespoons whole-wheat flour
1 cup vegetable stock
2 cups steamed pumpkin, puréed until very smooth
1 cup soy milk
$1/2$ teaspoon nutmeg
$1/4$ cup pepitas

1. In a medium soup pot, heat olive oil and sauté onion, salt, and pepper until onion is soft.

2. Stir in flour and cook for 2 to 3 minutes, stirring constantly. Slowly add vegetable stock and cook until mixture begins to thicken.

3. Add pumpkin, soy milk, and nutmeg. Heat through, then stir in pepitas. Serve hot or chill thoroughly and serve cold. Garnish with freshly grated nutmeg.

Carrot–Coconut Bisque

Serves 4

Basil adds a fresh green taste to this creamy, dairy-free soup, laced with the delicate undertones of nutmeg and shallots.

10 medium carrots, chopped
1 tablespoon olive oil
$^1/_2$ cup minced shallots
$^1/_2$ teaspoon white pepper
1 teaspoon sea salt
1 tablespoon whole-wheat flour
1 cup vegetable stock
1 $^1/_2$ cups light coconut milk
$^1/_2$ cup finely chopped basil (reserve a few sprigs for garnish)
$^1/_2$ teaspoon nutmeg

1. Steam carrots over medium heat until soft (about 7 to 10 minutes).

2. While carrots are steaming, heat olive oil in large soup pot and sauté shallots, pepper, and salt until shallots are translucent. Stir in flour and cook for 2 to 3 minutes. Slowly stir in stock and cook until mixture thickens.

3. Add carrots to stock mixture and purée until very smooth. Add coconut milk to carrot mixture and purée again until smooth.

4. Return to pot and stir in basil and nutmeg. Heat on low just until basil wilts (do not overcook—the coconut milk will lose its delicate flavor). Garnish with fresh sprigs of basil.

Roasted Red Pepper Sauce

Makes 2 cups

This smoky sauce is incredibly versatile—try it cold as a salad dressing, or heated and tossed with whole-grain pasta as a refreshing alternative to tomato sauce.

6 medium red peppers
2 tablespoons olive oil
$1/2$ teaspoon white pepper
1 teaspoon sea salt
$1/2$ cup finely chopped fresh basil

1. Place peppers on a baking sheet in a 400° oven for 30 to 45 minutes, turning several times until evenly charred on all sides. Wrap peppers in a damp towel to cool, then cut in half and remove stems and seeds.
2. Combine roasted peppers with olive oil, pepper, and salt. Purée until very smooth.
3. Add basil and blend well. Refrigerate to allow flavor to blend thoroughly, or serve hot.

Spicy Sweet Potato Unfries

Serves 6 to 8

Baked, not fried, this sweet and spicy appetizer or snack is a low-fat, nutrient-packed alternative to plain old French fries.

4 medium to large sweet potatoes, unpeeled
2 tablespoons olive oil
1 teaspoon sea salt
1 teaspoon white pepper
1 tablespoon curry powder
$1/2$ to 1 teaspoon cayenne pepper

1. Preheat oven to 375°.
2. Scrub sweet potatoes and cut in half. Cut each half into $1/4$-inch strips.
3. In a medium bowl, combine olive oil, salt, pepper, curry powder, and cayenne pepper. Mix well.
4. Add sweet potato strips to olive oil mixture and stir with hands until sweet potatoes are evenly coated. Spread on a cookie sheet and bake at 375° until tender. Serve hot.

Sautéed Peppers on Braised Radicchio
Serves 6

Sweet red and yellow peppers mix with the bitter flavors of radicchio and chicory and a delicate vinaigrette in this colorful combination salad or side dish.

3 red peppers
3 yellow peppers
1 tablespoon safflower oil
1 medium to large head radicchio, cut into 8 wedges
3 cups chicory, rinsed and torn into large pieces
1 tablespoon poppy seeds
$^1/_4$ cup raspberry vinegar
2 tablespoons walnut or almond oil
1 teaspoon sea salt

1. Core peppers and cut into $^1/_4$-inch strips. Steam just until barely tender, then rinse briefly under very cold water. Pat dry.

2. In a medium skillet, heat oil and lightly sauté radicchio and chicory just until wilted. Stir in poppy seeds, remove from pan and cool.

3. In a medium mixing bowl, combine vinegar, walnut or almond oil, and salt. Add peppers and stir until well coated. Place braised greens on a serving platter and arrange peppers on top. Chill or serve at room temperature.

Beets and Field Greens with Walnuts
Serves 4 to 6

Beets never had it so good! Even the fussiest feeders will love this sweet and tangy dish. Serve it well chilled as a salad, or alone for a light, super-healthy lunch.

$^1/_2$ cup chopped walnuts
2 cups cooked beets, peeled and julienned
2 cups mixed field greens, torn into medium-sized pieces
$^1/_4$ cup honey
$^1/_4$ cup raspberry vinegar
1 tablespoon safflower oil

1. Toast walnuts at 375° for about 8 minutes.

2. Combine beets, field greens, and toasted walnuts in large bowl.

3. Mix honey, vinegar, and oil in a small bowl. Blend until smooth and add to beet mixture, tossing well to coat completely. Chill thoroughly to allow flavors to blend.

Stuffed Red Peppers with Basil-Basmati Rice

Serves 6

Delicate basmati rice combines with basil, pine nuts, and wild mushrooms in this exotic take on stuffed peppers. A perfect party dish.

$^3/_4$ cup pine nuts
1 tablespoon olive oil
1 cup sliced wild mushrooms (chanterelles, morels, porcinis)
$^1/_2$ cup chopped shallots
2 cloves garlic, minced
1 teaspoon sea salt
1 teaspoon white pepper
6 large red peppers
3 cups cooked whole-grain basmati rice
$^1/_2$ cup finely chopped basil

1. Toast pine nuts at 375° for 5 minutes.
2. In a medium skillet, heat oil and sauté mushrooms, shallots, garlic, salt, and pepper until mushrooms are tender.
3. While mushrooms are sautéing, cut the tops off peppers and scoop out insides. Steam lightly in salted water for 2 to 3 minutes. Remove from heat, drain, and rinse with cold water. Pat dry.
4. Combine rice with toasted pine nuts and basil. Stir in mushroom mixture and blend well. Stuff each pepper with rice mixture.
5. Arrange peppers in lightly oiled casserole dish and bake at 375° for about 15 minutes, or until peppers are tender. Serve hot.

Orange Pepper Champagne Glaze

Makes 2 cups

This deliciously different, festive sauce is perfect as a glaze for fish dishes and as a light sauce on steamed greens or other vegetables for any special occasion.

3 yellow or orange peppers
1 teaspoon sea salt
$1/4$ teaspoon white pepper
1 tablespoon arrowroot
$1/2$ cup water
2 tablespoons honey
$1/4$ cup finely chopped basil
$1/2$ cup champagne

1. Core peppers, cut into chunks, and steam until soft. Let cool slightly.

2. Combine salt, pepper, arrowroot, water, and honey in a small saucepan. Heat to boiling, then simmer until sauce begins to thicken.

3. Purée peppers with honey mixture until very smooth. Return to pan, add basil and champagne, and heat through until sauce thickens. Serve hot.

Curried Yam Soup

Serves 6

Yummy yams pair up with curry and coconut milk in this hearty soup. Serve hot as a meal in itself or chilled as an intriguing appetizer.

1 tablespoon olive oil
1 medium yellow onion, diced
4 medium yams or sweet potatoes, unpeeled and cut into small cubes
2 cups vegetable stock
1 teaspoon sea salt
$1/2$ teaspoon white pepper
2 cups light coconut milk
$1/4$ cup finely chopped cilantro (reserve a few sprigs for garnish)

1. Heat oil in large soup pot and sauté onion until translucent.

2. Stir in yams, vegetable stock, salt, and pepper. Simmer, covered, until yams are tender.

3. Puree yam mixture until very smooth. Return to pot and stir in coconut milk and cilantro. Simmer 5 minutes to allow flavors to blend (be careful not to overcook—coconut milk loses its delicate flavor if cooked too long). Garnish with cilantro and serve hot, or chill thoroughly and serve cold.

RED/ORANGE/
YELLOW VEGETABLES

16

FISH

ZOOCHEMICALS
IN FISH

omega-3 fatty acids

vitamin A

Salmon Paté with Roasted Red Pepper and Chives

Makes 2 cups

A wonderful way to use leftover salmon. Smoky roasted pepper and fresh green chives make this a rich, satisfying, nutritious party appetizer.

2 small red peppers
1 pound cooked salmon
2 tablespoons lemon juice
1 small yellow onion, minced
3 garlic cloves, minced
$1/4$ cup finely chopped chives
$1/2$ cup soy mayonnaise

1. Place peppers on a baking sheet in a 400° oven for 30 minutes, turning several times until evenly charred on all sides. Wrap peppers in a damp towel to cool, then cut in half and remove stems and seeds.

2. Crumble salmon into a medium mixing bowl and sprinkle with lemon juice. Add onion, garlic, and chives, and mix well.

3. Briefly purée roasted peppers with mayonnaise until well mixed (don't blend too long—leave some chunks of pepper for texture).

4. Stir mayonnaise mixture into salmon and blend well. Refrigerate thoroughly until well chilled and flavors are completely combined.

Tuna Salad Niçoise with Avocado
Serves 4 to 6

Try this nouvelle take on the traditional French salad. Made with avocado and lots of tangy bitter greens, it's a fast and healthy lunchtime meal in itself, served with fresh, whole-grain bread.

1 medium bunch of arugula
1 small head of radicchio
2 medium heads of Belgian endive
1 pound cooked tuna
2 tablespoons lemon juice
1 teaspoon sea salt
$1/2$ teaspoon white pepper
1 medium avocado
1 cup diced cooked red potatoes, with skins on
$1/4$ cup capers
$1/4$ cup sliced black olives
$1/4$ cup red wine vinegar
2 tablespoons olive oil
$1/2$ teaspoon cracked black peppercorns
Several whole black olives for garnish

1. Wash greens well. Pat dry. Tear arugula and radicchio into bite-sized pieces, and slice endive $1/4$-inch thick. Toss together, and arrange on serving platter.

2. Crumble tuna into medium mixing bowl and sprinkle with lemon juice, salt, and pepper.

3. Slice avocado in half and remove seed. Peel and cut into $1/2$-inch cubes.

4. Combine potatoes, capers, and olives. In a small mixing bowl, combine wine vinegar and olive oil. Blend well. Stir into potato mixture.

5. On platter covered with greens, arrange tuna, potato mixture, and avocado chunks. Garnish with cracked black peppercorns and whole olives, and chill well before serving.

Hearty Fish Chowder

Serves 4 to 6

This creamy, dairy-free stew is packed with heart-healthy fish and lots of fresh vegetables—the ideal meal for cold winter days. Garnish with sprigs of parsley and a sprinkle of paprika and ground nutmeg.

1 tablespoon olive oil
1 small yellow onion, diced
2 garlic cloves, minced
1 teaspoon sea salt
2 tablespoons whole-wheat flour
3 cups vegetable stock
$\frac{1}{2}$ cup chopped carrots
$\frac{1}{2}$ cup sliced celery
1 cup diced potato, with skins on
$\frac{1}{2}$ cup fresh green peas
$\frac{1}{2}$ teaspoon black pepper
$\frac{1}{2}$ teaspoon nutmeg
$\frac{1}{2}$ pound swordfish
$\frac{1}{2}$ pound salmon
1 $\frac{1}{2}$ cups soy milk
$\frac{1}{4}$ cup red wine
2 tablespoons chopped fresh parsley

1. Heat oil in a large soup pot and sauté onion, garlic, and salt until onion is translucent. Add flour and cook for 2 to 3 minutes.

2. Slowly stir in vegetable stock and cook until mixture is thick and bubbly. Add carrots, celery, potato, peas, pepper, and nutmeg, and cook, covered, for 5 minutes.

3. While vegetables are cooking, wash fish thoroughly and cut into 1-inch cubes. Add to vegetable mixture and simmer, covered, until vegetables are tender and fish is flaky.

4. Stir in soy milk and heat through. Add red wine and parsley, and serve immediately.

Grilled Swordfish with Snow Peas and Water Chestnuts
Serves 4 to 6

Toasted sesame oil, spicy ginger, fresh snow peas, and crisp water chestnuts add an oriental flavor to this colorful fish dish. Serve over hot soba noodles with a simple salad of sliced cucumbers and diced tomatoes.

1 pound swordfish steaks
1 tablespoon toasted sesame oil
1 tablespoon light sesame oil
1 bunch scallions, thinly sliced
2 tablespoons freshly grated ginger
$1/2$ cup water chestnuts
1 tablespoon tamari
$1/2$ teaspoon black pepper
Up to $1/4$ cup water
1 cup snow peas, with stems removed
$1/2$ cup grated carrot
2 tablespoons sesame seeds

1. Wash swordfish steaks and cut into $1/2$-inch strips about 4 inches long.
2. Heat toasted sesame oil and light sesame oil in medium skillet. Sauté scallions and ginger until scallions are tender.
3. Add water chestnuts, tamari, pepper, and strips of fish. Sauté briefly, then add a little water and cook, covered, until fish is nearly done.
4. Stir in snow peas, grated carrot, and sesame seeds, and cook for 2 to 3 minutes longer, or until fish is cooked through and snow peas are bright green but still crisp. Serve over hot soba noodles.

Salmon-Stuffed Mushrooms

Serves 8 to 12

These tender little treats, made with flavorful salmon, basil, and red peppers, are great party appetizers or first-course dishes for special meals.

$^3/_4$ pound salmon
$^1/_2$ cup red wine
2 tablespoons olive oil
$^1/_2$ cup diced red onion
2 garlic cloves, minced
$^1/_2$ cup minced red pepper
$^1/_2$ cup finely chopped basil
1 teaspoon black pepper
1 teaspoon salt
$^1/_4$ cup bread crumbs
$^1/_2$ cup mozzarella-style soy cheese
2 dozen large mushroom caps
2 tablespoons finely chopped parsley

1. Wash salmon well and cut into cubes. Place in a medium skillet and poach in red wine until flaky.

2. Preheat oven to 375°.

3. While salmon is poaching, heat oil in a medium skillet. Sauté onion, garlic, red pepper, basil, black pepper, and salt until onion is soft.

4. Crumble cooked salmon with a fork and stir salmon and wine into onion mixture. Add bread crumbs and cheese.

5. Fill each mushroom cap with salmon stuffing. Arrange in a large, lightly oiled glass casserole, cover with foil, and bake at 375° for 15 minutes, or until mushrooms are tender and cheese is bubbly. Sprinkle with parsley and serve hot.

White Peppercorn Mako with Capers

Serves 4

This heart-healthy seafood version of steak au poivre is cooked up with capers and red wine for a rich but healthy dish. Just add steamed vegetables and whole-grain basmati rice for a fast, exotic meal.

4 small mako shark steaks (2 to 4 ounces each)
$1/4$ cup red wine
2 tablespoons lemon juice
2 garlic cloves, minced
1 tablespoon olive oil
1 tablespoon lightly crushed white peppercorns
$1/4$ cup capers

1. Wash steaks well. Pat dry and place on medium platter.
2. Combine red wine, lemon juice, garlic, and olive oil. Pour over fish steaks, coating each well. Marinate for 1 to 2 hours in refrigerator.
3. Sprinkle crushed peppercorns on a cutting board or covered surface. Coat both sides of each steak with peppercorns. Place steaks on a broiler pan and broil for 8 minutes. Sprinkle with capers and broil for 2 to 3 minutes longer, or until fish is done in center. Serve hot.

Seafood Etouffée

Serves 4 to 6

This nouvelle take on the classic New Orleans recipe is a piquant change of pace from ordinary fish dishes. Spicy and rich, it's still surprisingly low in fat. Serve with lots of brown rice.

1 tablespoon olive oil
3 garlic cloves, minced
$^{1}/_{2}$ cup chopped green pepper
$^{1}/_{2}$ cup chopped celery
$^{1}/_{2}$ cup chopped yellow onion
1 teaspoon sea salt
2 tablespoons whole-wheat flour
1 $^{1}/_{2}$ cups vegetable stock
$^{1}/_{2}$ pound tuna
$^{1}/_{2}$ pound sea bass
$^{1}/_{4}$ to $^{1}/_{2}$ teaspoon cayenne pepper
1 teaspoon black pepper
$^{1}/_{4}$ cup chopped fresh parsley (save a few sprigs for garnish)
2 very ripe tomatoes, cubed
2 bay leaves

1. In a heavy skillet (preferably cast-iron), heat olive oil and sauté garlic, green pepper, celery, onion, and salt until green pepper is tender. Add flour and cook for 3 to 5 minutes, or until flour turns golden brown.

2. Slowly add stock and stir until mixture is thick and bubbly.

3. While vegetables and stock are cooking, wash fish well and pat dry. Cut fish into $^{1}/_{2}$-inch cubes. In a medium mixing bowl, combine cayenne pepper and black pepper and mix well. Add fish cubes and stir to coat well.

4. Stir fish into vegetable mixture. Add parsley, tomatoes, and bay leaves, and simmer for 10 to 15 minutes, or until fish is flaky. Remove bay leaves and serve etouffée hot over rice, garnished with parsley.

Smoked Salmon Salad
with Lemon–Honey Cucumbers
Serves 6

Fresh green cucumbers, lightly marinated in a sweet and tangy glaze, are a marvelous complement to smoky salmon. Served on a bed of bitter chicory, pungent arugula, and bright red radicchio, it's a colorful salad for any occasion.

$1/4$ cup lemon juice
$1/4$ cup honey
$1/2$ teaspoon sea salt
2 medium cucumbers, peeled and cut into $1/4$-inch slices
1 small head of chicory
1 small bunch of arugula, with stems removed
1 small head radicchio
1 pound smoked salmon, thinly sliced
2 teaspoons finely chopped fresh parsley

1. In a medium mixing bowl, combine lemon juice, honey, and salt. Stir in cucumber slices to coat well, and let marinate for 1 hour in refrigerator.

2. While cucumbers are marinating, immerse chicory, arugula, and radicchio completely in ice-cold water to remove all sand and dirt. Drain, rinse again, and pat dry. Tear into bite-size pieces and arrange on decorative serving platter.

3. Arrange fish on bed of mixed lettuce. Place marinated cucumbers on top of fish and drizzle with remaining marinade. Sprinkle with parsley for garnish and chill before serving.

Tuna–Olive Paté

Makes 2 cups

Fresh tuna is the best, but if you're in a pinch, canned tuna is an adequate substitute. Serve as a savory spread with crackers, or as a dip with chips.

1 pound cooked tuna
2 tablespoons lemon juice
1 bunch scallions, finely sliced, with green tops
1 medium tomato, diced
$^1/_2$ cup sliced black olives
$^1/_2$ cup soy mayonnaise
$^1/_2$ teaspoon white pepper

1. Crumble tuna into a medium mixing bowl and sprinkle with lemon juice. Add scallions, diced tomato, and olives, and mix well.
2. Stir mayonnaise and white pepper into tuna mixture and blend well. Refrigerate thoroughly until well chilled and flavors are completely combined.

Grilled Mako with Orange Pepper Champagne Glaze

Serves 4

Hearty (and heart-healthy) grilled mako shark steaks team up with an exotic pepper glaze for a festive and nutritious meal. Serve with Almond Rice with Green Peas (page 177) and a colorful array of steamed veggies.

4 small mako shark steaks (2 to 4 ounces each)
3 garlic cloves, minced
$^1/_2$ teaspoon black pepper
1 $^1/_2$ cups Orange Pepper Champagne Glaze (see page 159)

1. Rinse steaks well and pat dry. Rub with garlic and black pepper, and grill over hot coals (or broil in oven) for about 7 minutes, or until tender and flaky.
2. While fish is cooking, heat glaze over low just until warmed through.
3. Remove fish to serving platter and drizzle with glaze. Serve hot.

17

NUTS AND SEEDS

**PHYTOCHEMICALS
IN NUTS AND SEEDS**

lignins

phenols (including ellagic acid)

isoflavones

vitamin E

fatty acids

Cumin-Roasted Walnuts
Makes 2 cups

Heart-healthy walnuts make a great alternative to empty-calorie snacks. This savory sweet-and-salty combination, with the pungent flavors of cumin and garlic and a delicate hint of honey, makes an outstanding party appetizer. Or use as a garnish to spice up salads and almost any dish.

2 cups coarsely chopped walnuts
6 cloves garlic
2 tablespoons olive oil
2 tablespoons ground cumin
1 tablespoon cumin seed
1 teaspoon sea salt
2 tablespoons honey

1. Toast walnuts at 375° for 8 to 10 minutes.
2. Peel garlic cloves and squeeze through garlic press (to make peeling cloves easier, drop into boiling water for 30 seconds—skins will slip off easily).
2. Heat oil in medium skillet. Sauté garlic until golden. Stir in ground cumin, cumin seed, salt, and honey
4. Add toasted walnuts to skillet. Stir well to coat.
5. Spread evenly on baking sheet and bake at 375° for 20 minutes, or until golden. Cool thoroughly.

Sesame–Herb Bread

Makes one loaf

Crunchy white and black sesame seeds team up in this savory quick bread, packed with whole-grain nutrition and lots of fresh green herbs.

2 $1/2$ cups whole-wheat flour
$1/2$ teaspoon baking soda
1 teaspoon aluminum-free baking powder
1 teaspoon salt
1 $1/2$ cups water
$1/2$ cup silken tofu
$1/4$ cup finely chopped fresh sage
$1/4$ cup finely chopped fresh basil
$1/4$ cup finely chopped fresh parsley
$1/4$ cup light sesame seeds
$1/4$ cup black sesame seeds
2 tablespoons safflower oil

1. Preheat oven to 350°.
2. Combine flour, baking soda, baking powder, and salt in a medium bowl. Mix well to combine.
3. Purée water and tofu until very smooth. Stir tofu mixture into flour and blend well. Stir in sage, basil, parsley, light sesame seeds, and black sesame seeds.
4. Coat loaf pan with oil and turn batter into pan. Bake at 350° for 45 minutes to 1 hour, or until completely cooked in the center (until a toothpick comes out clean).
5. Cool for 20 to 30 minutes, turn out of pan and serve hot.

Sunny Sprouted Avocado Salad
Serves 6

Rich, creamy avocados combine with field greens and a crunchy combination of sprouted beans and seeds in this colorful, festive salad. A light summer lunch all by itself, or serve as the first course with a soup dinner.

2 ripe avocados
1 cup sprouted sunflower seeds
$^1/_2$ cup sprouted lentils
$^1/_2$ cup sprouted mung beans
1 small head oak leaf lettuce
1 small bunch arugula
1 small head raddichio

Dressing
$^1/_4$ cup raspberry vinegar
$^1/_4$ cup walnut or almond oil
$^1/_4$ cup natural raspberry jam or preserves
1 teaspoon sea salt
1 teaspoon white pepper
Edible flowers for garnish (optional)

1. Cut avocados in half. Remove pit, peel, and cut into cubes.

2. Combine sprouted sunflower seeds, sprouted lentils, and sprouted mung beans in a medium mixing bowl. Add avocados to mixing bowl.

3. Completely immerse lettuce, arugula, and radicchio in ice-cold water to remove all sand and dirt. Drain, rinse again, and pat dry. Tear into bite-size pieces and arrange on decorative serving platter.

4. To make dressing, combine vinegar, oil, raspberry preserves, salt, and pepper. Mix well until thick and smooth.

5. Add dressing to avocado and sprout mixture and toss gently. Turn onto platter with lettuces. Chill thoroughly before serving and garnish with edible flowers.

To make sprouts: Soak sunflower seeds, lentils, and mung beans overnight in separate jars. Drain, rinse thoroughly, drain well, and let sit until sprouted. Sunflower seeds can be used as soon as small nubs begin to appear at the tips (about 12 hours). Lentils can be used when small, white sprouted tips begin to appear (12 to 24 hours). Mung beans are ready when about $^1/_4$-inch white tips have appeared (12 to 24 hours). Be careful not to oversprout—the beans and seeds become bitter.

Easy Almond Milk

Makes 4 cups

A delicious, dairy-free alternative to milk. This delicate beverage can be sweetened with honey or rice syrup, and flavored with natural vanilla or almond extract. Serve with cereal or fruit for breakfast, or over ice for a refreshing summer drink.

1 cup blanched almonds
3 cups water
Natural vanilla or almond extract (optional)
Honey or rice syrup (optional)

1. Purée almonds and water in a food processor at high speed for 5 minutes.
2. Strain almond mixture through damp cheesecloth, squeezing out excess liquid. Discard almonds left in cheesecloth.
3. Stir in vanilla or almond extract and honey or rice syrup if desired. Chill thoroughly and keep refrigerated.

Vanilla–Berry Butter

Makes 2 cups

The subtle taste of vanilla accompanies fresh fruit and tahini for a creamy, dairy-free alternative to butter. Drizzle over pancakes, waffles, or muffins for breakfast, or use as a sandwich filling on Walnut-Oat Bread (page 123).

$^1/_2$ cup natural applesauce
$^1/_4$ cup natural apple or blueberry juice
$^1/_2$ cup tahini
$^1/_4$ cup honey
1 tablespoon vanilla
$^1/_2$ cup raspberries or blueberries

1. Combine applesauce and juice in a medium mixing bowl.
2. Stir in tahini, honey, and vanilla, and mix well.
3. Add berries and crush with the back of a wooden spoon. Beat by hand until creamy and smooth. Refrigerate to let flavors blend. Serve chilled, or heat just until soft to use as a thick syrup.

Peanut Soba Noodles

Makes 4 to 6 servings

This oriental classic is a colorful change of pace from regular pasta dishes. Crisp snow peas, bright red peppers, and crunchy water chestnuts add texture and extra flavor to this simple supper dish.

1 pound dry soba noodles
1 tablespoon light sesame oil
1 small yellow onion, diced
2 garlic cloves, minced
1 teaspoon sea salt
$1/2$ teaspoon white pepper
$1/2$ cup diced red pepper
$1/2$ cup sliced water chestnuts, rinsed and drained well
$1/4$ cup smooth peanut butter
$1/4$ cup rice syrup
$1/4$ cup hot water
1 cup snow peas, with stems removed
$1/2$ cup finely chopped peanuts

1. In a large soup pot, boil 2 quarts of water with a pinch of salt. Add noodles and cook until just tender. Drain and return to pan.

2. While noodles are cooking, heat sesame oil in a medium skillet. Sauté onion, garlic, salt, and white pepper until onion is translucent. Add diced red pepper and water chestnuts, and simmer until red pepper is tender.

3. In a small mixing bowl, combine peanut butter, rice syrup, and hot water. Blend until smooth and creamy.

4. Add peanut mixture and snow peas to onion mixture in skillet and heat through until snow peas are just tender and sauce is thick and bubbly.

5. Combine peanut sauce with noodles in soup pan and mix until noodles are well coated. Stir in chopped peanuts and serve hot, or chill thoroughly and serve cold.

Sesame–Ginger Shrimp
Serves 4 to 6

Bright carrots and a splash of sake add color and flavor to this savory medley of spicy ginger, pungent shiitakes, and tender shrimp. Serve with brown rice and braised greens with a splash of rice vinegar for a tasty, oriental-style meal.

2 tablespoons light sesame oil
1 small red onion, diced
1 cup sliced shiitake mushrooms
$1/2$ teaspoon sea salt
$1/4$ cup freshly grated ginger
2 tablespoons tamari
2 tablespoons honey
$1/4$ cup sake
1 tablespoon arrowroot
1 cup shredded carrot
$1/2$ cup sesame seeds
1 pound medium shrimp, peeled, washed, and deveined

   1. Heat oil in medium skillet. Sauté onion, mushrooms, and salt until mushrooms are limp.

   2. Add ginger, tamari, honey, sake, and arrowroot to mushroom mixture and cook until mixture begins to thicken.

   3. Stir in shredded carrot, sesame seeds, and shrimp. Sauté until shrimp is opaque (about 5 minutes). Serve hot.

Almond Rice with Green Peas

Serves 6

Tired of plain old brown rice? Try this colorful, crunchy dish with bright green peas and the nutty taste and texture of almonds as a side dish to any meal.

$1/2$ cup slivered almonds
2 cups brown basmati rice
4 cups vegetable stock
1 cup fresh green peas
1 teaspoon sea salt
$1/2$ teaspoon black pepper
2 tablespoons almond oil

1. Toast almonds in a 375° oven for 5 minutes.
2. Combine rice and stock in large saucepan. Bring to boil, then reduce to a simmer and cook, covered, about 30 minutes.
3. Stir in peas and cook, covered, for 15 minutes longer, or until peas are soft.
4. Gently stir in toasted almonds, salt, pepper, and almond oil. Serve hot as a side dish.

Double Delicious Pesto

Makes 3 to 4 cups

A decidedly different take on the traditional pesto dish. This flavorful sauce uses walnuts and almonds in addition to pine nuts for a super-nutty taste.

3 cups finely chopped basil
$1/4$ cup olive oil
$1/4$ cup pine nuts
$1/4$ cup finely chopped walnuts
$1/4$ cup almonds
3 cloves garlic, minced
1 teaspoon sea salt
1 teaspoon white pepper

Combine all ingredients in a blender and purée until very smooth, adding water as needed to make a thick paste. Serve hot over pasta or vegetables.

Nice and Nutty Veggie Burgers

Serves 4 to 6

Chock full of nuts and savory mushrooms, with the delicate undertones of tahini, these tasty burgers are a great way to use leftover beans and grains. Perfect for fast and easy dinners, served with Beets and Field Greens with Walnuts salad (p. 157).

$^1\!/_2$ cup walnuts
2 cups cooked beans (lentils, garbanzos, pintos, or a combination of all)
2 tablespoons tahini
1 tablespoon olive oil
$^1\!/_2$ cup diced onion
$^1\!/_2$ cup sliced mushrooms
1 teaspoon sea salt
$^1\!/_2$ teaspoon black pepper
$^1\!/_2$ cup sunflower seeds
1 cup millet, rice, or other cooked grains

1. Toast walnuts at 375° for 8 to 10 minutes. Let cool and chop finely.
2. Purée beans and tahini until smooth, adding water as needed.
3. In a medium skillet, heat olive oil and sauté onion, mushrooms, salt, and pepper until mushrooms are limp. Let cool.
4. Combine bean mixture with mushroom mixture in a medium mixing bowl. Mix well, and stir in walnuts and sunflower seeds. Add grains and use hands to mix until well blended. Chill for 1 to 2 hours.
5. Shape burger mixture into patties about 3 to 4 inches wide. Sauté, grill, or broil until done in center (about 5 minutes per side).

18

BEANS

PHYTOCHEMICALS
IN BEANS

isoflavonoids

phytate

fiber (including lignins)

folic acid

Three-Bean Indian Dal

Serves 6 to 8

A combination of beans and celery seed gives a new flavor twist to this traditional Indian stew—and it's a great way to use leftover beans. Served with whole-wheat pita bread, it's the perfect one-pot meal for cold winter nights.

2 tablespoons olive oil
1 medium red onion, diced
$\frac{1}{2}$ cup sliced celery
4 cloves garlic, minced
1 small green pepper, diced
1 teaspoon sea salt
$\frac{1}{2}$ teaspoon white pepper
1 tablespoon celery seed
1 tablespoon ground cumin
2 teaspoons coriander
2 tablespoons freshly grated ginger
2 large tomatoes
3 cups water
1 cup cooked lentils
1 cup cooked black beans
1 cup cooked garbanzo beans
$\frac{1}{4}$ cup chopped cilantro (reserve a few whole sprigs for garnish)

1. Heat oil in large soup pot and sauté onion, celery, garlic, green pepper, salt, and white pepper until green pepper is tender. Add celery seed, ground cumin, coriander, and ginger and sauté for 3 minutes longer.

2. Core tomatoes and dice. Add to onion and pepper mixture, and sauté until tomatoes are soft and juicy.

3. Add water, lentils, black beans, garbanzo beans, and cilantro to soup pot and simmer, covered, for 10 to 15 minutes. Serve hot, garnished with cilantro.

Basil–Lentil Stew

Serves 4 to 6

Lots of fresh green basil and fresh vegetables add color—and a delicate, unexpected flavor—to traditional lentil soup. Try it for a super-simple, one-dish dinner.

1 tablespoon olive oil
1 medium yellow onion, diced
1 cup sliced shiitake mushrooms or button mushrooms
2 cloves garlic, minced
1 teaspoon sea salt
1 teaspoon black pepper
1 medium green pepper, diced
1 medium red pepper, diced
$^1/_2$ cup chopped carrots
$^1/_2$ cup cubed red potatoes, with skins on
$^1/_2$ cup chopped basil
4 cups vegetable stock
1 cup dry lentils

1. Heat oil in large soup pot and sauté onion, mushrooms, garlic, salt, and black pepper until onions are translucent.

2. Add green pepper, red pepper, carrots, and potatoes to soup pot. Sauté for 3 to 5 minutes.

3. Stir in basil, stock, and lentils. Bring to a boil, then reduce heat and simmer, covered, for about 30 to 40 minutes, or until vegetables are tender and lentils are soft.

Mexican Bean Salad

Serves 4 to 6

A tasty take on three-bean salad with a spicy, south-of-the-border flavor. Perfect for picnics, light lunches, or as an easy party dish.

1 tablespoon safflower oil
$^1/_4$ cup finely diced hot green pepper
2 cloves garlic, crushed
$^1/_2$ cup finely chopped yellow onion
1 teaspoon sea salt
1 teaspoon black pepper
$^1/_2$ cup diced green pepper
1 cup diced tomatoes
$^1/_2$ teaspoon cayenne
1 teaspoon chili powder
$^1/_4$ cup chopped cilantro
1 cup cooked black beans
1 cup cooked kidney beans
1 cup cooked pinto beans
$^1/_4$ cup red wine vinegar

1. In a medium skillet, heat oil and sauté hot green pepper, garlic, onion, salt, and black pepper until onion is translucent.

2. Stir in diced green pepper, tomatoes, cayenne, chili powder, and cilantro, and heat just until cilantro begins to wilt.

3. Turn tomato and pepper mixture into a medium mixing bowl. Add black beans, kidney beans, pinto beans, and vinegar. Mix well and chill thoroughly before serving.

Lentil–Garlic Paté

Makes 4 cups

This protein-packed, low-fat alternative to meat patés has a nutty, garlicky flavor that goes with everything from crackers to crudités.

1 cup lentils
3 to 4 cups water
2 tablespoons olive oil
6 garlic cloves, minced
$1/4$ cup chopped shallots
1 cup silken low-fat tofu
1 teaspoon white pepper
1 teaspoon sea salt
$1/4$ cup finely chopped basil

1. Rinse lentils well and place in a heavy pan with water. Bring to a boil, cover, reduce heat, and simmer for 30 minutes, or until soft. Add water as needed.

2. While lentils are cooking, heat oil in a medium skillet and sauté garlic and shallots briefly (about 2 to 3 minutes).

3. Mash tofu in a medium bowl and stir in pepper and salt. Add garlic and shallots.

4. Drain any excess water from lentils and add to tofu mixture. Purée until very smooth. Stir in basil and chill thoroughly to let flavors combine. Serve in a decorative bowl as a dip for pita wedges or raw, fresh vegetables.

Simon-and-Garfunkel Black Bean Soup

Serves 6 to 8

Lots of parsley, sage, rosemary, and thyme add a fresh green taste to this simple soup with black beans and lots of vegetables. Serve with a bitter greens salad, hot sourdough bread, and the appropriate music.

1 tablespoon olive oil
1 small red onion, chopped
1 teaspoon sea salt
$1/2$ teaspoon black pepper
$1/2$ cup chopped carrots
$1/2$ cup diced tomato
$1/2$ cup chopped celery
$1/2$ cup diced potato, with skins on
3 cups vegetable stock
2 cups cooked black beans
$1/4$ cup finely chopped fresh parsley
$1/4$ cup finely chopped sage
$1/4$ cup finely chopped rosemary
$1/4$ cup finely chopped thyme

1. Heat oil in a large soup pot and sauté onion, salt, and pepper until onion is translucent.

2. Stir in carrots, tomato, celery, and potato, and sauté until tomato pieces begin to give up their juices. Add vegetable stock and simmer, covered, until vegetables are tender.

3. Add beans, parsley, sage, rosemary, and thyme, and heat through until flavors are well blended (about 5 to 10 minutes).

White Bean Soup with Sage

Serves 6

Lightly browned sage, red wine, and a hint of honey bring out the delicate flavor of white beans in this creamy, memorable soup.

1 tablespoon olive oil
1 leek, thinly sliced (including green top)
2 garlic cloves, minced
1 teaspoon sea salt
$^1/_2$ teaspoon white pepper
$^1/_2$ cup finely chopped sage (reserve a few whole sprigs for garnish)
1 tablespoon whole-wheat flour
4 cups vegetable stock
1 tablespoon honey
2 cups cooked white beans
1 cup cooked brown rice or other grains
$^1/_4$ cup red wine

1. Heat oil in a large soup pot and sauté sliced leek, garlic, salt, and pepper until leek is tender. Add sage and sauté until sage begins to brown.

2. Stir in flour and cook for 2 to 3 minutes. Slowly stir in vegetable stock and honey, and simmer until mixture begins to thicken.

3. Add cooked beans, cooked rice, and wine, and heat through until beans are soft. Serve in individual bowls garnished with sprigs of fresh sage.

Hot and Spicy Hummus

Makes 4 cups

Lots of spices and herbs add extra flavor to this pungent version of a traditional Middle Eastern favorite. Serve at room temperature as a spread on warm pita bread or for dipping raw veggies.

3 cups cooked garbanzo beans
1 cup tahini
$1/4$ cup lemon juice
3 cloves garlic, crushed
$1/2$ teaspoon white pepper
1 teaspoon sea salt
1 teaspoon ground cumin
$1/2$ teaspoon hot red pepper flakes
$1/2$ teaspoon cayenne pepper
$1/2$ teaspoon black pepper
$1/4$ cup finely diced hot green peppers
Red pepper slices for garnish

1. Purée garbanzo beans, tahini, and lemon juice until smooth, adding water as needed to make a creamy mixture. Pour into medium mixing bowl.

2. Add garlic, white pepper, salt, cumin, pepper flakes, cayenne, black pepper, and hot green peppers to garbanzo bean mixture. Stir well.

3. Chill to allow flavors to blend. Serve as an appetizer, garnished with red pepper slices.

Baked Chickpea Loaf

Serves 6 to 8

This colorful, cheesy bean casserole combines garbanzo beans with rosemary, lots of fresh vegetables, and creamy millet or hearty brown rice—a wonderful, dairy-free way to use leftover beans and grains.

2 tablespoons olive oil
$^1/_2$ cup diced red pepper
$^1/_2$ cup diced green pepper
$^1/_2$ cup chopped carrots
$^1/_2$ cup sliced shiitake mushrooms
1 medium red onion, thinly sliced
2 tablespoons whole-wheat flour
$^1/_2$ cup red wine
$^1/_2$ cup vegetable stock or water
1 cup firm low-fat tofu
1 teaspoon sea salt
1 teaspoon black pepper
$^1/_4$ cup fresh rosemary, finely chopped
2 cups cooked garbanzo beans
2 cups cooked millet or short-grain brown rice
1 cup cheddar-style soy cheese

1. Preheat oven to 375°.
2. Heat oil in a medium skillet. Sauté red pepper, green pepper, carrots, mushrooms, and onion until carrots are tender.
3. Stir in flour and cook for 2 to 3 minutes longer. Slowly stir in red wine and stock, and mix until smooth.
4. Purée tofu, salt, and pepper until very smooth. Stir in rosemary and combine with cooked vegetables in medium mixing bowl.
5. Add garbanzo beans and millet or rice to tofu and vegetable mixture. Mix well.
6. Spread mixture into a lightly oiled casserole and sprinkle with soy cheese. Cover lightly with foil and bake at 375° for 20 minutes. Remove foil and bake for 5 to 10 minutes longer, or until cheese is bubbly.

Curried Mung Beans
Serves 4 to 6

When's the last time you had mung beans? Can't remember? Then try this spicy dish, made with a delicate coconut-curry sauce and tender little beans. Serve as a side dish with rice, or as a light lunch with fresh, hot bread to soak up curry sauce.

1 cup mung beans
4 cups water
1 cup coconut milk
1 medium yellow onion, diced
1 teaspoon sea salt
$\frac{1}{2}$ cup vegetable stock
2 tablespoons dried curry mix
1 teaspoon white pepper
1 teaspoon cumin
1 teaspoon coriander
Cilantro for garnish

1. Soak mung beans overnight. Rinse well and place in a large soup pot with water. Bring to a boil and cook for 30 minutes, or until tender.

2. While beans are cooking, combine coconut milk, onion, and sea salt in medium mixing bowl. Let stand 10 minutes, then mix well with hands, squeezing juice from onion.

3. Stir stock into coconut milk mixture and blend well. Add curry mix, white pepper, cumin, and coriander.

4. Add coconut milk and stock mixture to beans and heat through gently (don't overcook—excess heat will destroy the delicate flavor of coconut milk).

Garnish with sprigs of cilantro and serve hot.

Azuki Beans and Greens

Serves 4 to 6

A simple, flavorful way to use these traditional Japanese beans. While often overlooked, they're packed with nutrition and flavor. A great side dish or first course.

1 cup azuki beans
4 cups water
1 tablespoon light sesame oil
1 teaspoon toasted sesame oil
$1/2$ cup diced yellow onion
2 garlic cloves, minced
1 teaspoon black pepper
1 tablespoon sesame seeds
1 pound kale, collard greens, or chard
$1/4$ cup tamari

1. Soak beans overnight. Drain soaking water, rinse well, and combine in large soup pot with water. Bring to a boil, cover, and let simmer for 1 hour, or until beans are tender.

2. While beans are cooking, heat sesame oil and toasted sesame oil in a large skillet. Sauté onion, garlic, pepper, and sesame seeds until onion is translucent and seeds begin to turn golden.

3. Wash greens well, remove stems, and chop into bite-sized pieces. Add to skillet with onion mixture and stir to coat with oil. Add tamari and cook just until greens begin to wilt.

4. Drain any excess water from beans and add to greens mixture in skillet. Simmer for 10 minutes, until beans are soft and greens are tender.

19

ONIONS AND GARLIC

**PHYTOCHEMICALS
IN ONIONS AND GARLIC**

organosulfur compounds

(including allylic sulfides)

flavonoids (including quercetin)

coumarin

ellagic acid

Garlic-Stuffed Red Peppers

Serves 6

Water chestnuts and ginger, along with an ample amount of pungent garlic and a hint of honey, add an oriental flair to this nutritious, tasty dish.

1 tablespoon light sesame oil
$^1/_2$ cup finely chopped scallions
6 garlic cloves, minced
1 cup sliced water chestnuts, rinsed well and drained
1 cup snow peas, with stems removed
1 tablespoon tamari
2 tablespoons freshly grated ginger
6 medium red peppers
2 cups cooked brown rice
$^1/_4$ cup sesame seeds
2 tablespoons honey
2 tablespoons rice vinegar

1. Preheat oven to 375°.

2. In a medium skillet, heat sesame oil and sauté scallions and garlic until scallions are translucent.

3. Stir in water chestnuts, snow peas, tamari, and ginger, and sauté briefly (about 1 to 2 minutes).

4. Cut the tops off the red peppers and scoop out seeds. Rinse well and pat dry.

5. Add rice, sesame seeds, honey, and vinegar to the water chestnut mixture and mix well. Stuff each pepper with rice filling. Bake at 375° for about 15 minutes, or until peppers begin to get soft.

Garlic Hummus with Roasted Red Peppers

Makes 4 cups

The smoky flavor of roasted red pepper, pungent shallots, black olives, and extra garlic add a special taste to this twist on the traditional Middle Eastern dish. Perfect as a spread on warm, whole-wheat pita bread with lots of alfalfa sprouts.

2 medium red peppers
3 cups cooked garbanzo beans
1 cup tahini
$^1/_4$ cup lemon juice
5 cloves garlic, crushed
$^1/_4$ cup minced shallots
$^1/_2$ teaspoon white pepper
1 teaspoon sea salt
$^1/_2$ cup sliced black olives

1. Place peppers on a baking sheet in a 400° oven for 30 to 45 minutes, turning several times until evenly charred on all sides. Wrap peppers in a damp towel to cool, then cut in half and remove stems and seeds.

2. While peppers are roasting, purée garbanzo beans, tahini, and lemon juice until smooth, adding water as needed to make a creamy mixture. Pour into medium mixing bowl.

3. Add garlic, shallots, white pepper, and sea salt. Mix well.

4. Cut red peppers into strips and purée briefly (about 30 seconds) with hummus mixture. Stir in olives. Chill thoroughly to allow flavors to blend.

Creamy Garlic Sauce
Makes 1 1/2 cups

This rich, dairy-free sauce is so versatile it can be served almost any way—heat it up and drizzle over vegetables or fish, toss with pasta, or chill and serve as a pungent dressing on green salads.

1 tablespoon olive oil
8 cloves garlic, crushed
1 teaspoon salt
$\frac{1}{2}$ teaspoon white pepper
1 tablespoon flour
$\frac{1}{2}$ cup vegetable stock
1 cup soy milk

1. Heat oil in a medium skillet. Sauté garlic, salt, and pepper until garlic is soft.

2. Stir in flour and cook for two to three minutes. Slowly blend in vegetable stock and soy milk, cooking on low until mixture is thick and creamy.

3. Serve hot, or chill thoroughly.

Garlic-Baked Jalapeño Bites

Serves 8 to 12

Hot and spicy, these south-of-the-border taste-treats make perfect party appetizers. Serve with crackers and lots of cold beverages!

2 tablespoons olive oil
8 garlic cloves, minced
$1/2$ cup minced red onion
$1/2$ teaspoon sea salt
$1/2$ cup finely diced red pepper
$1/4$ cup pine nuts
1 cup grated mozzarella-style soy cheese
12 large jalapeño peppers

1. Heat oil in medium skillet. Sauté garlic, onion, salt, and red pepper until garlic is golden.

2. While garlic is sautéing, spread pine nuts on a cookie sheet and toast at 375° for about 5 minutes.

3. Stir toasted pine nuts into garlic mixture. Remove from heat. Add soy cheese and stir until well mixed.

4. Slice each pepper lengthwise and stuff with cheese mixture. Bake at 375° in a glass casserole for about 10 minutes, or until peppers are tender and cheese is bubbly.

French Onion Soup

Serves 4 to 6

A fresh, light take on traditional French onion soup, this tasty concoction uses sweet Vidalia onions, soy cheese, and a hint of sage for a fresh, green taste.

2 tablespoons olive oil
4 medium Vidalia onions, sliced
4 garlic cloves, minced
$1/2$ teaspoon sea salt
$1/2$ teaspoon black pepper
6 cups vegetable stock
$1/4$ cup red wine
$1/4$ cup finely chopped fresh sage
4 to 6 $1/4$-inch slices whole-wheat baguette, toasted
1 cup grated mozzarella-style soy cheese

1. Heat oil in a large soup pot. Sauté onions, garlic, salt, and pepper until onions are golden.
2. Add stock, cover and simmer for 20 to 30 minutes.
3. Stir in red wine and sage, and cook, uncovered, for 5 to 10 minutes longer.
4. Pour soup into oven-proof bowls. Top each serving with a slice of toasted bread and sprinkle with cheese. Bake at 375° until cheese is bubbly. Serve immediately.

Tarragon–Leek Soup

Serves 4 to 6

A rich dairy-free stew, brimming with tomatoes, flavorful leeks, fresh tarragon, and a whisper of honey and red wine. Perfect for snowy winter days.

1 tablespoon olive oil
2 medium leeks, sliced with green tops
2 garlic cloves, minced
1 teaspoon sea salt
1 tablespoon whole-wheat flour
$\frac{1}{2}$ cup diced tomatoes
$\frac{1}{2}$ cup tomato juice
4 cups vegetable stock
1 tablespoon honey
$\frac{1}{4}$ cup finely chopped fresh tarragon
$\frac{1}{4}$ cup red wine

1. Heat oil in large soup pot. Sauté leeks, garlic, and salt until garlic is golden.
2. Stir in flour and cook for 2 to 3 minutes longer, stirring constantly.
3. Slowly stir in tomatoes, tomato juice, and stock, and cook until mixture thickens. Add honey and tarragon, and simmer, covered, for 10 minutes.
4. Add red wine and serve immediately.

Parsley–Garlic Pitas
Serves 8

Whole-wheat pitas are the perfect vehicle for a fresh-tasting garlic–parsley spread with olive oil—a refreshing change of pace from regular garlic bread. Serve hot with soups and salads, or as an appetizer for any meal.

4 large whole-wheat pitas
4 tablespoons olive oil
6 garlic cloves, minced
1 teaspoon black pepper
$1/2$ cup finely chopped parsley

1. Cut each pita in half and gently separate.
2. Heat oil in medium skillet and sauté garlic and pepper until garlic is golden. Stir in parsley and cook for 1 to 2 minutes longer.
3. Drizzle garlic and olive oil mixture on pita halves and bake at 350° for 5 to 7 minutes, or until pitas are warmed through.

Baked Garlic Cloves
Serves 6

This pungent spread is a heart-healthy, fat-free alternative to butter. Spread on warmed whole-grain breads for a delicious addition to any meal.

6 medium to large whole garlic cloves
1 tablespoon olive oil
1 teaspoon sea salt
2 tablespoons finely chopped fresh oregano
2 tablespoons finely chopped fresh basil

1. Place garlic cloves on a cookie sheet and drizzle with olive oil.
2. Bake at 400° for about 20 to 30 minutes, or until garlic is soft and fragrant. Sprinkle with salt, oregano, and basil, and serve hot.

Fennel with Red Onions
Serves 4

The often overlooked fennel bulb has a distinctive anise flavor that's complemented by red onions and basil in this savory side dish.

2 medium fennel bulbs
1 tablespoon olive oil
1 medium red onion, sliced
2 garlic cloves, minced
1 teaspoon sea salt
$^1/_2$ teaspoon white pepper
$^1/_4$ cup finely chopped fresh basil

1. Wash fennel well and cut each bulb into eighths.
2. Heat oil in medium skillet and sauté onion, garlic, salt, and pepper until onion is just tender.
3. Stir in fennel and mix to coat well with olive oil. Lower heat and sauté gently until fennel is tender. Add basil and cook for 2 to 3 minutes longer.

Wild Mushroom Sauté with Leeks
Serves 4 to 6

A real taste-treat for mushroom lovers. Leeks and lots of garlic combine with basil and smoky wild mushrooms in this hearty, tantalizing appetizer.

1 tablespoon olive oil
4 cups sliced mushrooms (morels, chanterelles, porcinis, shiitakes, or other)
2 cups sliced leeks, with green tops
1 teaspoon sea salt
$^1/_2$ teaspoon white pepper
4 garlic cloves, minced
$^1/_2$ cup finely chopped fresh basil

1. Heat oil in a medium skillet and sauté mushrooms, leeks, salt, pepper, and garlic until mushrooms are tender.
2. Stir in basil, and cook just until basil wilts. Serve immediately as a side dish or appetizer.

APPENDIX:
FINDING YOUR PHYTOS

THIOLS

Broccoli
Brussels sprouts
Cabbage
Cauliflower
Garlic
Mustard
Onions
Radishes

CAROTENOIDS

Apricots
Cantaloupe
Carrots
Citrus fruits
Greens (mustard, kale, collard, turnip, spinach, etc.)
Guava
Papaya
Parsley
Red grapefruit
Strawberries
Tomatoes

Watermelon
Winter squash
Yams/sweet potatoes

PHENOLICS

Apples
Beans
Berries
Broccoli
Brussels sprouts
Cabbage
Carrots
Citrus fruits
Cucumbers
Eggplant
Flaxseed
Grapes
Green tea and black tea
Peanuts
Peas
Pomegranates
Rosemary
Soybeans

TERPENOIDS

Apricots
Basil
Broccoli
Cabbage
Cantaloupe
Carrots
Cucumbers
Citrus fruits
Eggplant
Greens (mustard, kale, collard, turnip, spinach, etc.)
Licorice
Mangos
Mint
Parsley
Peppers
Red grapefruit
Summer squash
Tomatoes
Watermelon
Winter squash
Yams/sweet potatoes

ORGANIC ACIDS

Beans and legumes
Lima beans
Peanuts
Rice bran
Sesame seeds
Soybeans
Whole grains

RETINOIDS/RETINOL

Cod-liver oil
Swordfish
Whitefish

EFAS

Cold-water fish/shellfish (zoochemicals)
Flaxseed
Nuts
Seeds

INDOLES

Broccoli
Cabbage
Brussels sprouts
Greens (mustard, kale, collard, turnip, spinach, etc.)

ISOPRENOIDS/VITAMIN E/ TOCOPHEROLS/ TOCOTRIENOLS

Nuts and seeds
Rice-bran oil
Unprocessed or minimally processed oils
Wheat germ
Whole grains

VITAMIN C/ASCORBIC ACID

Berries
Broccoli
Citrus fruits
Greens (mustard, kale, collard, turnip, spinach, etc.)
Parsley
Peppers
Tomatoes

Source: Marcia Zimmerman & Associates, Westlake Village, CA; Anthony Almada, Myogenix, Palo Alto, CA

NOTES

Introduction

1. M. L. Y. Jenkins, "Research Issues in Evaluating 'Functional Foods'," *Food Technology* 47 (1993):5, 76-79; divisions of foods and function as cited in the *Federal Register*, vol. 58, no. 3 (1993).

Chapter 1: Coming to Terms with Nutraceuticals

1. M. Cole, "When Food Meets Medicine," *Food Review*, June-July 1991, 15-17.
2. A. Bendich and J. A. Olson, "Biological Actions of Carotenoids," *FASEB Journal* 3 (1989): 1927-1932; A. Bendich, *Journal of Nutrition* 119 (1989):112-115; R. S. Parker, "Carotenoids in Human Blood and Tissues," *Journal of Nutrition* 119 (1989):101-104.
3. P. Nair et al., *American Journal of Clinical Nutrition* 40 (1984):4, 927-930.

Chapter 2: The Changing of the Nutritional Guard

1. A. B. Caragay, "Cancer-Preventing Foods and Ingredients," *Food Technology*, April 1992, 65-68.
2. S. J. Olshansky, B. A. Carnes, and C. Cassel, "In Search of Methuselah: Estimating the Upper Limits to Human Longevity," *Science* 250 (1990):634-639.
3. D. M. Tucker et al., "Nutrition Status and Brain Function in Aging," *American Journal of Clinical Nutrition* 52 (1990):93-102; R. G. Cutler, "Antioxidants and Aging," *American Journal of Clinical Nutrition* 53 (1991):3735-3795.
4. Michelle Stacey, *Consumed: Why Americans Love, Hate, and Fear Food*, New York: Simon & Schuster, 1994.

Chapter 3: The Best Defense

1. Study results from "HealthFocus on U.S. Consumers Survey," conducted by HealthFocus Inc., Des Moines, Iowa, 1994.

2. T. R. Covington et al., eds., *Handbook of Nonprescription Drugs*, Washington, D.C.: American Pharmaceutical Association, 1993, 283-311.

3. K. J. Rothman et al., "Teratogenicity of High Vitamin A Intake," *New England Journal of Medicine* 333 (1995):21, 1369-1415.

4. Nancy Bruning, ed., *The Natural Health Guide to Antioxidants*, New York: Bantam Books, 1994; A. Bendich, "Safety Issues Regarding the Use of Vitamin Supplements," *Annals of the New York Academy of Sciences* 669 (1992):300-310; M. Cohen and A. Bendich, "Safety of Pyridoxine: A Review of Human and Animal Studies," *Toxicology Letters* 34 (1986):129-139; A. Bendich and M. Cohen, "Vitamin B$_6$ Safety Issues," *Annals of the New York Academy of Sciences* 585 (1990):321-330.

5. M. Wahlqvist, "Changes in Serum Carotenoids in Subjects with Colorectal Adenomas after 24 Mo of Beta-Carotene Supplementation," *American Journal of Clinical Nutrition* 6 (1994):936-994.

6. L. J. Machlin, "Free Radical Tissue Damage and the Protective Role of Antioxidant Nutrients," *Twentieth Samuel Brody Memorial Lecture*, Special Report 414 Agr. Exp. Station, Columbia, Mo.: University of Missouri, 1988.

Chapter 4: Live Longer, Look Younger, Feel Better

1. Carper, Jean, *Food: Your Miracle Medicine*, New York: HarperCollins Publishers Inc., 1993, 256-257; Salaman, Maureen, *Foods That Heal*, Menlo Park, Ca: MKS, Inc., 1989, 287.

2. U.S. Dept. of Health & Human Services, "The Surgeon General's Report on Nutrition and Health," Washington, D.C.: U.S. Government Printing Office, 1995.

3. L. A. G. Ries et al., eds., *SEER Cancer Satistics Review, 1973-1991: Tables and Graphs*, Bethesda, Md.: National Cancer Institute, 1994, NIH Pub. No. 94-2789.

4. G. Colditz et al., "Increased Green and Yellow Vegetable Intake and Lowered Cancer Death in an Elderly Population," *American Journal of Clinical Nutrition* 41 (1985):1; Kedar N. Prasad, *Vitamins in Cancer Prevention and Treatment*, Rochester, Vt.: Healing Arts Press, 1994.

5. R. Harris et al., "A Case Controlled Study of Dietary Carotene in Men with Lung Cancer and Men with Other Epithelial Cancer," *Nutrition and Cancer* 15 (1991): 63-68; T. Hirayama, "Diet and Cancer," *Nutrition and Cancer* 1 (1979):67-81; R. B. Shekelle et al., "Dietary Vitamin A and Risk of Cancer in the Western Electric Study," *Lancet* 2 (1981):1185-1190.

6. J. A. Wylie-Rossett et al., "Influence of Vitamin A on Cervical Dysplasia and Carcinoma In Situ," *Nutrition and Cancer* 6 (1984):49-57; R. W. C. Harris et al., "Cancer of the Cervix Uteri and Vitamin A," *British Journal of Cancer* 53 (1986):653-659; K. Brock et al., "Nutrients in Diet and Plasma and Risk of In Situ Cervical Cancer," *Journal of the National Cancer Institute* 80 (1988):580-585.

7. L. Packer, "Protective Role of Vitamin E in Biological Systems," *American Journal of Clinical Nutrition*, suppl., 53 (1991):1, 1052s-1053s; P. Knekt et al., "Serum Vitamin E and Risk of Cancer Among Finnish Men During a 10-Year Follow-up," *American Journal of Epidemiology* 127 (1988):28-41.

8. S. S. Mirvish, "Effects of Vitamins C and E on N-Nitroso Compound Formation, Carcinogenesis, and Cancer," *Cancer* 58 (1986):1842-1850; N. J. Wald et al., "Plasma Retinol, Beta Carotene, and Vitamin E Levels in Relation to the Future Risk of Breast Cancer," *British Journal of Cancer* 49 (1984):321-324.

9. Shari Lieberman and Nancy Bruning, *The Real Vitamin and Mineral Book,* Garden City Park, N.Y.: Avery Publishing Group, 1990, 116, 246.

10. U. S. Department of Health and Human Services, *The Surgeon General's Report on Nutrition and Health,* Washington, D.C.: U.S. Government Printing Office, 1988.

11. Committee on Diet, Nutrition, and Cancer, National Research Council, *Cancer, Diet and Health: Implications for Reducing Chronic Risk,* Washington, D.C.: National Academy Press, 1989, 593-605.

12. J. Liu et al., "Inhibition of 7,12-Dimethylbenz(a)anthracene-Induced Mammary Tumors and DNA Adducts by Garlic Powder," *Carcinogenesis* 13 (1992):1847-1851; D. S. B. Hoon et al., "Modulation of Cancer Antigens and Growth of Human Melanoma by Aged Garlic Extract," *Garlic and Biology in Medicine: Proceedings of the First World Congress on the Health Significance of Garlic and Garlic Constituents,* Irvine, Calif.: Nutrition International Co., 1990; J. Pinto et al., "Effects of Aged Garlic Extract on Cultured Human Breast Cancer Cells," unpublished manuscript, 1993; W. J. Blot, "Garlic in Relation to Cancer in Human Populations," *Garlic and Biology in Medicine: Proceedings of the First World Congress on the Health Significance of Garlic and Garlic Constituents,* Irvine, Calif.: Nutrition International Co., 1990.

13. M. J. Stampfer et al., "A Protective Study of Vitamin E Supplementation and Risk of Coronary Disease in Women," American Heart Association Scientific Session, November 17, 1992.

14. M. Boogaerts et al., "Protective Effect of Vitamin E on Immune Triggered, Granulocyte Mediated Endothelial Injury," *Thrombosis Haemostas* (Stuttgart) 51 (1984):89-92; M. Steiner, "Effect of Vitamin E on Platelet Function and Thrombosis," *Agents and Actions* 22 (1987):357-358; K. C. Srivastava, "Vitamin E Exerts Antiaggregatory Effects Without Inhibiting the Enzymes of the Arachidonic Acid Cascade in Platelets," *Prostaglandins Leukotrienes and Medicine* 21 (1986):177-185; A. Szczeklik et al., "Dietary Supplementation with Vitamin E in Hyperlipoproteinemias: Effects on Plasma Lipid Peroxides, Antioxidant Activity, Prostacyclin Generation, and Platelet Aggregability," *Thrombosis Haemostas (Stuttgart)* 54 (1985):425-430.

15. The first study examined 87,000 nurses in the Nurses' Health Study at Brigham and Women's Hospital and found that those women with the highest consumption of dietary beta-carotene had a 22 percent lower risk of heart attack. A second study, the Physician's Health Study—involving 20,000 physicians at the Harvard School of Public Health in conjunction with Brigham and Women's Hospital, conducted by Charles Hennekens, M.D., and Meir Stampfer, M.D.—examined the effects of beta-carotene in a group of men with a history of heart disease. The study is still under way, but preliminary data suggest that the group of more than 300 men who took 50 mg of beta-carotene every other day were half as likely to die of heart disease as those who did not take supplemental beta carotene. J. A.

Manson et al., "Antioxidants and Cardiovascular Disease," *Journal of the American College of Nutrition* 12 (1993):426-432.

16. P. Jaques, "Effects of Vitamin C on High-density Lipoprotein Cholesterol and Blood Pressure," *Journal of the American College of Nutrition* 11 (1992):139-144; E. Greenberg et al., "A Clinical Trial of Antioxidant Vitamins to Prevent Colorectal Adenoma," *New England Journal of Medicine* 331 (1991):141-147.

17. Robert I-San Lin, "Phytochemicals and Antioxidants," in Israel Goldberg, ed., *Functional Foods: Designer Foods, Pharmafoods, Nutraceuticals,* New York: Chapman & Hall, 1994; Chez Giang Medical University, *Medical Science Report,* Pharmaceutical section 6 (1972):13; Wu Han Army General Hospital, *New Medical Science* 1 (1973):13.

18. B. Stavric et al., "Flavonoids in Foods: Their Significance for Nutrition and Health," in *Lipid Soluble Anitoxidants,* S. H. Ong Augustine and Lester Packer, eds., Basel: Birkhauser Verlag, 1992.

19. "Obesity," *Nutrition Week* 25 (1995):7, American Heart Association, AHA Scientific/Medical Position Paper, January 1995.

20. P. Rous, "The Influence of Diet on Transplanted and Spontenous Tumors," *Journal of Experimental Medicine* 20 (1914):433-451; A. Tannenbaum et al., "The Genesis and Growth of Tumors . . . Effects of Varying the Proportion of Protein (Casein) in the Diet," *Cancer Research* 9 (1949):162-173; D. F. Birt, "Fat and Calorie Effects on Carcinogenesis at Sites Other Than the Mammary Gland," *American Journal of Clinical Nutrition* 45 (1987):203-209; D.F. Birt et al., "Influence of Diet and Calorie Restriction on the Initiation and Promotion of Skin Carcinogenesis in the Sencar Mouse Model," *Cancer Research* 51 (1991):1851-1854.

21. Robert H. Garrison and Elizabeth Somer, *The Nutrition Desk Reference,* New Canaan, Conn.: Keats Publishing, 1985, 159.

22. The Framingham Heart Study, based in Framingham, Massachusetts, has followed more than 800 men since the mid-1950s. Some of the studies have found that men with blood-pressure levels greater than 160 over 95 were two to three times more likely to suffer stroke or heart disease and that none of the subjects in the study with a cholesterol level lower than 150 milligrams per deciliter had a heart attack.

23. A study of 722 Eastern Finnish men without a history of hyptertension found that high blood levels of vitamin C and selenium were related to lower blood pressure: J. T. Salonen, "Dietary Fats, Antioxidants, and Blood Pressure," *Annals of Medicine* 23 (1991):295-298. In another study, a survey of more than 11,000 Americans found that those with the highest blood pressure levels had the lowest consumption of vitamin C: D. A. McCarron et al., "Blood Pressure and Nutrient Intake in the United States," *Science* 224 (1984):1392-1398. This inverse relationship between blood pressure and vitamin C has been confirmed by a number of research findings.

24. K. P. West et al., "Vitamin A and Infection: Public Health Implications," *Annual Review of Nutrition* 9 (1989):63-86.

25. A. Bendich, "Carotenoids and Immunity," *Clinical and Applied Nutrition* 1 (1991):45-51; M. Alexander et al., "Oral Beta-Carotene Can Increase the Number of OKT4+ Cells in Human Blood," *Immunology Letters* 9 (1985):221-225.

NOTES

26. *1984-1985 Yearbook of Nutritional Medicine*, New Cannan, Conn.: Keats Publishing, 1985, 126; P. Knekt et al., "Serum Vitamin E and Risk of Cancer Among Finnish Men," *American Journal of Epidemiology* 127 (1988):41; M. Meydani, "Vitamin E Health Benefits," *Lancet* 345 (1995):170-76.

27. One study, in which healthy young adults were given 1,000 to 3,000 mg per day of vitamin C for three weeks, showed increased T-cell activity: R. Anderson et al., "The Effect of Increasing Weekly Doses of Ascorbate on Certain Cellular and Humoral Immune Functions in Normal Volunteers," *American Journal of Clinical Nutrition* 33 (1980):71-76. Another study showed that 10,000 mg of vitamin C per day in young adults increased lymphocyte proliferation and antibody responses: R. S. Panush et al., "Modulation of Certain Immunologic Responses by Vitamin C III Potentiation of In Vitro and In Vivo Lymphocyte Responses," *International Journal for Vitamin and Nutrition Research*, suppl., 23 (1982):35-47. Subjects in a University of Arizona study who took only 500 mg of vitamin C per day showed a 50 percent increase in blood levels of glutathione, another powerful water-soluble antioxidant that helps the body ward off infection and detoxify drugs and other potentially toxic compounds: C. S. Johnson, *American Journal of Clinical Nutrition* 58 (1993):103-105.

28. M. C. Goldschmidt et al., "The Effect of Ascorbic Acid Deficiency on Leukocyte Phagocytosis and Killing of *Actinomyces viscosus*," *International Journal for Vitamin and Nutrition Research* 58 (1988):326-333.

29. Nancy Bruning, ed., *The Natural Health Guide to Antioxidants*, New York: Bantam Books, 1994; Sheldon Saul Hendler, *The Doctors' Vitamin and Mineral Encyclopedia*, New York: Simon & Schuster, 1991.

30. A study done by Dr. Kenneth Cochran at the University of Michigan in 1960 suggests that an antiviral carbohydrate substance in shiitake mushrooms called lentinan stimulates the immune system, boosts T-cell activity, and encourages the immune system to produce interleukin-1, an immune-cell "hormone" that helps prevent tumor growth.

31. K. J. A. Davies et al., "Free Radicals and Tissue Damage Produced by Exercise," *Biochemical and Biophysical Research Communications* 107 (1982):1198-1205.

32. One study conducted at Columbia University by researcher Stanley Fahn showed that high levels of vitamin E (3,200 IU per day) and vitamin C (3,000 mg per day) helped to slow the progression of Parkinson's disease. In another study, vitamin E seemed to prevent the death of nerve cells that can lead to Alzheimer's: *News from the Salk Institute*, July 31, 1992; reported in Michael Granberry, "Breakthrough in Alzheimer's Is Reported," *Los Angeles Times*, July 31, 1992. Another study found that even slight deficiencies of carotenoids can slow mental function: James Penland, USDA's Grand Forks Human Nutrition Research Center.

CHAPTER 5: THE DYNAMIC DOZEN

1. Edward Behr, *The Artful Eater*, New York: The Atlantic Monthly Press, 1992.
2. Jean Carper, *Stop Aging Now!*, New York: HarperCollins, 1995, 170.

3. P. Talalay et al., Baltimore, Md.: Johns Hopkins University, "The Proceedings of the National Academy of Sciences," Sept. 12, 1995, v. 92, no. 19, 8846; K. Napier, "Green Revolution," *Harvard Health Letter* 20 (1995):9.

4. R. K. Tiwari et al., "Selective Responsiveness of Human Breast Cancer Cells to Indole-3-Carbinol, a Chemopreventive Agent," *Journal of the National Cancer Institute* 86 (1994):126.

5. J. W. Erdman, Jr., "Control of Serum Lipids with Soy Protein," *New England Journal of Medicine* 333 (1995):313. In another study, a review of almost 40 clinical trials showed that substituting soy protein for animal protein helped decrease blood-cholesterol levels and blood-lipid levels. An intake of 25 grams of soy protein per day resulted in a decrease of 9 milligrams per deciliter of cholesterol, while an intake of 50 grams per day led to a reduction of 17 milligrams, and 75 grams resulted in a reduction of 26 milligrams: J. W. Anderson et al., "Meta-analysis of the Effects of Soy Protein Intake on Serum Lipids," *New England Journal of Medicine* 333 (1995):276.

6. T. Akiyama et al., "Use and Specificity of Genistein as an Inhibitor of Protein-Tyrosine Kinases," *Methods in Enzymology* 201 (1991):362-370; T. Fotsis et al., "Genistein, a Dietary Derived Inhibitor of In Vitro Angiogenesis," *Proceedings of the National Acadamy of Sciences, USA* 90 (1993):2690-2694; Mark Messina, Ph.D., and Virginia Messina, R.N., *The Simple Soybean and Your Health*, New York: Avery Publishing Group, 1994.

7. Some researchers believe that excess iron may increase the risk of heart disease: J. L. Beard, "Are We at Risk for Heart Disease Because of Normal Iron Status?" *Nutrition Reviews* 51 (1993):112-115; R. B. Lauffer, *Iron Balance*, New York: St. Martins Press, 1991. Other research has pointed to the free-radical inhibiting actions of phytate and their benefit in treating a variety of diseases, as well as the role of protease inhibitors in soy products: Mark Messina, Ph.D., and Virginia Messina, R.N., *The Simple Soybean and Your Health*, New York: Avery Publishing Group, 1994.

8. L. U. Thompson et al., "Phytic Acid and Minerals: Effect on Early Markers of Risk for Mammary and Colon Carcinogenesis," *Carcinogenesis* 12 (1991):2041-2045; E. Graf et al., "Suppression of Colonic Cancer by Dietary Phytic Acid," *Nutrition and Cancer* 19 (1993):9.

9. H. L. Newmark, "Plant Phenolics as Inhibitors of Mutational and Precarcinogenic Events," *Canadian Journal of Physiology and Pharmacology* 65 (1987):461-466; H. L. Newmark, "A Hypothesis for Dietary Components as Blocking Agents of Chemical Carcinogenesis: Plant Phenolics and Pyrolle Pigments," *Nutrition and Cancer* 6 (1984):58-70.

10. Low-fat diets in concert with high-fiber intake have been shown to lower LDL cholesterol levels: P. Marckmann et al., "Low-Fat, High-Fiber Diet Favorably Affects Several Independent Risk Markers of Ischemic Heart Disease," *American Journal of Clinical Nutrition* 59 (1994): 4, 935. In one study, the risk of colon or rectal cancer was reduced by more than 30 percent by increasing fiber intake to 39 grams per day: "Reducing Colon Cancer Risk," *Medical World News* 34 (1993):56. In

another analysis of dozens of epidemiologic studies, fiber-rich diets were found to help protect against colorectal cancer: J. W. Anderson et al., "Health Benefits and Practical Aspects of High-Fiber Diets," *American Journal of Clinical Nutrition*, suppl., 59 (1994):1242s-1247s.

11. In one study, men with a high intake of cereal fiber had a lower rate of heart disease than those with a low intake of cereal fiber: J. N. Morris et al., "Diet and Heart: A Postscript," *British Medical Journal* 2 (1977):1307-1314. Other studies have found that obesity may be controlled with high-fiber diets, through a variety of mechanisms: diets rich in fiber slow gastric emptying and increase the feeling of fullness, decrease blood concentrations of insulin—which helps lower appetite, may increase metabolism, can stimulate the release of peptides that reduce food consumption, and take longer to eat, thereby increasing the feeling of fullness: J. W. Anderson, "Dietary Fiber and Human Health," *Journal of Horticultural Science* 25 (1990):1488-1495. Fiber may also help control diabetes—a review of 53 studies examining the effects of fiber supplements in diabetics showed that fiber supplements improved glycemic control and lowered cholesterol levels in 67 percent of the cases studied: J. W. Anderson et al., "Treatment of Diabetes with High Fiber Diets," in G. A. Spiller, ed., *Handbook of Dietary Fiber in Human Nutrition*, Boca Raton, Fla.: CRC Press, 1993; J. W. Anderson et al., "Health Benefits and Practical Aspects of High-Fiber Diets," *American Journal of Clinical Nutrition*, suppl., 59 (1994):1242s-1247s.

12. In a study conducted by Dr. James Cerda at the University of Florida, patients with high cholesterol were given about half an ounce of grapefruit pectin capsules per day and showed an 8 percent reduction in total cholesterol levels after about four months: Jean Carper, *The Food Pharmacy*, New York: Bantam Books, 1988, 214-215. A modified version of citrus pectin can ward off prostate cancer in rats, according to a study by researcher Kenneth Pienta, M.D., and colleagues. Several other studies have shown that citrus pectin can inhibit the growth of cancer cells and enhance immunity: K. Pienta et al., *Journal of the National Cancer Institute* 87 (1995):5.

13. J. F. Scheer, "Latest on Cataracts," *Bestways*, September 1986, 20.

14. D. Sharp, "East Meets West on Stomach Cancer," *Lancet* 345 (1995):1041.

15. Researchers from Tufts University in Boston and the Framingham Heart Study in Framingham, Massachusetts, found that the consumption of greens can reduce heart disease, primarily because of the folic-acid content in greens. In examining more than 1,000 patients over a three-year period, the researchers found that of those participants with the most severe cases of atherosclerosis, 43 percent of the men and 34 percent of the women also had elevated homocysteine blood levels and that their diets were lacking in folic acid: "Green Vegetables Reduce Risk of Heart Disease," *Medical Update* 18 (1995):1.

16. One animal study showed that spinach helped lower overall cholesterol levels: N. Iritani et al., "Effect of Spinach and Wakame on Cholesterol Turnover in the Rat," *Atherosclerosis* 15 (1972):87-92. In another study of more than 50,000 British nurses,

those consuming the highest amounts of vitamin A reduced their risk of cataracts by 39 percent, and the protective effect was the strongest for women who ate spinach: S. E. Hankinson et al., "Nutrient Intake and Cataract Extraction in Women: A Prospective Study," *British Medical Journal* 305 (1992):335. Another study showed that Americans who ate lutein-rich greens such as spinach two to four times a week were almost half as likely to develop macular degeneration: *Tufts University Diet and Nutrition Letter* 12 (1995):11.

17. Jean Carper, *Stop Aging Now!*, New York: HarperCollins 1995; Garry G. Duthie, and Katrina M. Brown, "Reducing the Risk of Cardiovascular Disease," in Israel Goldberg, ed., *Functional Foods: Designer Foods, Pharmafoods, Nutraceuticals,* New York: Chapman & Hall, 1994, 25-27.

18. Jean Carper, *Food: Your Miracle Medicine,* New York: Harper Perennial, 1994, 356-358. *Journal of Urology* 131 (1984):1013; *Wisconsin Medical Journal* 61 (1962):282; *Southwestern Medicine* 47 (1966):17; *Nursing Times* 87 (1991):36.

19. According to some studies, guava fruit may lower blood-cholesterol levels by as much as 10 percent, by virtue of its high fiber content: K. Napier, "Green Revolution," *Harvard Health Letter* 20 (1995):9. Fruits also contain ample amounts of vitamin C, as well as certain phenolic acids, substances that have been shown to prevent cancer by inhibiting cancer-cell growth: T. Tanaka et al., "Chemoprevention of Digestive Organs Carcinogenesis by Natural Product Protocatechic Acid," *Cancer* 75 (1995):1433. Flavonoids in fruits have been shown to help prevent heart disease and reduce cancer risk: M. G. Hertog et al., "Flavonoid Intake and Long-term Risk of Coronary Heart Disease and Cancer in the Seven Countries Study," *Archives of Internal Medicine* 155 (1995):381. Other research suggests that ellagic acid in grapes, raspberries, and strawberries may help prevent cancer: M. Ternus, "Fresh Fruit: Sweet Way to Get Vitamins, Fiber, and More," *Environmental Nutrition* 18 (1995):5.

20. Researchers examined almost 2,000 men for a 13-year period and found a strong correlation between lower blood-carotenoid concentrations and a higher rate of heart disease: D. L. Morris et al., *Journal of the American Medical Association* 272 (1994):1439-1441.

21. One study of almost 3,000 men over a 12-year period showed that lower blood levels of A, C, E, and carotenoids were related to a higher rate of death from cancer: J. A. Hattner, "Reduce Your Risk of Cancer," *USA Today* 123 (1995):72.

22. D. A. Leaf et al., "Incorporation of Dietary Fatty Acids into the Fatty Acids of Human Adipose Tissue and Plasma Lipid Classes," *American Journal of Clinical Nutrition* 62 (1995):68.

23. LDL-cholesterol levels tend to increase with a decreased consumption of fish oils: S. M. Kleiner, "Savoring Seafood," *Executive Health's Good Health Report* 29 (1993):6-7; Lewis Harrison, *Making Fats and Oils Work for You,* New York: Avery Publishing Group, 1990. EPA and DHA can help diminish the negative effects of a diet high in fat. EPA can also help relieve migraine headaches and has been shown to relieve rheumatoid arthritis pain: Lewis Harrison, *Making Fats and Oils Work for You.*

24. Omega-3 fatty acids may have beneficial effects against breast cancer, according to a study conducted by Dr. David P. Rose from the American Health Foundation in

Valhalla, New York: "Inhibition of Breast Cancer Progression with Omega-3 Fatty Acids," *Cancer Biotechnology Weekly*, April 17, 1995, 10. Omega-3s have also been shown to prevent or slow the growth of cancer tumors in general: G. Fernandes et al., "Modulation of Breast Cancer Growth in Nude Mice by Omega-3 Lipids," *World Review of Nutrition and Dietetics* 66 (1991):488-503; and diets high in omega-3 fatty acids have beneficial effects against several types of malignant tumors: W. T. Cave, "Omega-3 Fatty Acid Diet Effects on Tumorigenesis in Experimental Animals," in A. P. Simopoulos, R. R. Kifer, R. E. Martin, and S. M. Barlow, eds., *Health Effects of Omega-3 Polyunsaturated Fatty Acids in Seafoods*, vol. 66, Basel: Karger, 1991, 74-86.

25. T. A. Mori et al., "Effects of Varying Dietary Fat, Fish, and Fish Oils on Blood Lipids in a Randomized Controlled Trial in Men at Risk of Heart Disease," *American Journal of Clinical Nutrition* 59 (1994):1060-1068.

26. Healthy men were fed two cholesterol-lowering diets—one that used walnuts as the source of fat and another that used other types of fat. The group of men who consumed walnuts showed a drop in average cholesterol from 182 to 160: J. Sabate et al., "Effects of Walnuts on Serum Lipid Levels and Blood Pressure in Normal Men," *New England Journal of Medicine* 328 (1993):603.

27. K. Napier, "Green Revolution," *Harvard Health Letter* 20 (1995):9.

28. In a 1992 study, researchers at Loma Linda University in California examined the lifestyles of more than 31,000 Seventh-day Adventists to determine factors behind their low rates of heart disease and cancer: J. Sabat, *Archives of Internal Medicine* 152 (1992):1416.

29. J. Shugar et al., "Effect of Ellagic and Caffeic Acids on Covalent Binding of Benzo(a)pyrene to Epidermal KNA of Mouse Skin on Organ Culture," *International Journal of Biochemistry* 16 (1984):571-573; R. L. Chang et al., "Effect of Ellagic and Hydroxylated Flavonoids on the Tumorigenicity of Benzo(a)pyrene on Mouse Skin and in the Newborn Mouse," *Carcinogenesis* 6 (1985):1127-1133.

30. K. Napier, "Green Revolution," *Harvard Health Letter* 20 (1995):9.

31. In one study, less than half a cup of pumpkin seeds per day reduced nighttime urination by 95 percent, urgency of urination by 81 percent, and frequency of urination by 73 percent: Jean Carper, *Food: Your Miracle Medicine*, New York: HarperCollins, 1993.

32. J. Hurley and S. Schmidt, "It's Bean Great," *Nutrition Action Healthletter* 20 (1993):12.

33. M. P. Zupke, "A Hill of Beans Amounts to a Lot of Nutrition," *Environmental Nutrition* 16 (1993):2.

34. One study found that people who eat beans on a regular basis have a 97 percent lower risk of developing pancreatic cancer: P. K. Mills et al., "Dietary Habits and Past Medical History as Related to Fatal Pancreas Cancer Risk Among Adventists," *Cancer* 61 (1988):2578-2585. In another study, the bean consumption and cancer rate of 15 countries was compared, and the analysis revealed that bean consumption was associated with decreased risks of colon, breast, and prostate cancer: P. Correa, "Epidemiologic Correlations between Diet and Cancer Frequency," *Cancer Research* 41 (1981):3685-3689.

35. Lignins, also called phytoestrogens, have been shown to have estrogen-like prop-

erties and to help regulate estrogen levels and activity. High consumption of foods rich in lignins may reduce the risk of certain types of cancer that are related to estrogen levels, especially breast cancer: H. A. Adlercreutz et al., "Effect of Dietary Components, Including Lignins and Phytoestrogens on Enterohepatic Circulation and Live Metabolism of Estrogens and on Sex Hormone Binding Globulin," *Journal Steroid Biochemistry* 27 (1987):1135-1144; T. Hirano et al., "Antiproliferative Activity of Mammalian Lignin Derivative against Human Breast Carcinoma Cell Line, ZR-75-1," *Cancer Investigator* 8 (1990):595-601. Lignins and isoflavonoids may also have a chemopreventive effect on cancers of the male reproductive system.

36. H. Adlercreutz, "Does Fiber Rich Food Containing Animal Lignin Precursors Protect Against Both Colon and Breast Cancer? An Extension of the 'Fiber Hypothesis'," *Gastroenterology* 86 (1984):761-764; H. Adlercreutz, "Western Diet and Western Disease: Some Hormonal and Biochemical Mechanisms and Association," *Scandinavian Journal Clinical Lab Investigation* 50 (1990):3-23.

37. Other compounds in beans and legumes include phytates, which can help prevent certain types of intestinal cancer. Epidemiological studies have shown a lower rate of cancer among people who consume higher quantities of beans, perhaps in part by the action of phytates. E. Graf and J. W. Eaton, "Suppression of Colonic Cancer by Dietary Phytic Acid," *Nutrition and Cancer* 19 (1993):11-19.

38. Michelle Stacey, *Consumed: Why Americans Love, Hate, and Fear Food,* New York: Simon & Schuster, 1994; F. S. Goulart, "Garlic and Onion: Nature's 100-Watt Bulbs," *Total Health* 17 (1995):36.

39. R. I. S. Lin, "First World Congress on the Health Significance of Garlic and Garlic Constituents," August 1990.

40. K. Napier, "Green Revolution," *Harvard Health Letter* 20 (1995):9.

41. In large studies of people in China and Italy, people who regularly consumed high quantities of garlic and onions demonstrated a lower risk of stomach cancer: E. Dorant et al., "Garlic and Its Significance for the Prevention of Cancer in Humans: A Critical Review," *British Journal of Cancer* 67 (1993):424-429.

42. K. A. Steinmetz et al., "Vegetables, Fruit, and Colon Cancer in the Iowa Women's Health Study," *American Journal of Epidemiology* 139 (1994):1-15.

43. Garlic can lower blood-cholesterol levels by as much as 10 to 21 percent, according to Jonathan Isaacsohn, M.D., of Yale University, speaking at a seminar, "Garlic: An International Dialogue on Cardiovascular Benefits," April 21, 1991, in New York.

44. In one study, garlic significantly lowered overall cholesterol levels while raising levels of HDL cholesterol. In a related study, garlic decreased LDL cholesterol and overall cholesterol levels: "Garlic," *Lawrence Review of Natural Products,* April 1994.

45. F. S. Goulart, "Garlic and Onion: Nature's 100-Watt Bulb," *Total Health* 17 (1995):36.

CHAPTER 6: THE NEW ANTIOXIDANTS AND NOVEL COMPOUNDS

1. H. McCord, "Going for the 'French Factor': Do Flavonoids in Red Wine and Foods Promise Health 'Affairs of the Heart'?" *Prevention* 47 (1995):74-80.

2. Studies have shown that light drinkers have a lower risk of heart disease than

those who don't drink at all: A. L. Klatsky, "Can a Drink a Day Keep a Heart Attack Away?" *Patient Care* 29 (1995):39-50. One study examining flavonoid intake in seven different countries found that the higher the intake of flavonoids, the lower the death rate from heart disease: M. G. L. Hertog et al., "Flavonoid Intake and Long-term Risk of Coronary Heart Disease and Cancer in the Seven Countries Study," *Archives of Internal Medicine* 155 (1995): 318-386.

3. One landmark study showed that people who drank two glasses of red wine a day for two weeks had a lower oxidation level of LDL cholesterol than when they drank no wine, and white wine actually caused higher levels of LDL-cholesterol oxidation, a biological phenomenon that increases the risk of developing atherosclerosis or heart disease: B. Furhman et al., "Consumption of Red Wine with Meals Reduces the Susceptibility of Human Plasma and Low-Density Lipoprotein to Lipid Peroxidation," *American Journal of Clinical Nutrition* 61 (1995):549-554. Other human studies have confirmed these results, demonstrating that phenolic compounds in red wine inhibit LDL oxidation and that the antioxidant effect of red wine is greater than that of vitamin E: E. N. Frankel et al., "Inhibition of Oxidation of Human Low-Density Lipoprotein by Phenolic Substances in Red Wine," *Lancet* 341 (1993):454-457.

4. "Grape Juice and Wine Share Secret of Lowering Cholesterol," *Environmental Nutrition* 15 (1992):7.

5. "Lower Your Cholesterol with Grape Juice," *East West Natural Health* 22 (1992):16.

6. R. D. Moore et al., "Moderate Alcohol Consumption and Coronary Heart Disease: A Review," *Medicine* 65 (1986):242-267; L. A. Friedman et al., "Coronary Heart Disease Mortality and Alcohol Consumption in Framingham," *American Journal of Epidemiology* 24 (1986):481-489.

7. Jean Carper, *Food: Your Miracle Medicine,* New York: HarperCollins, 1993.

8. A. L. Klatsky et al., "Alcohol Consumption and Blood Pressure," *New England Journal of Medicine* 296 (1977):1194-1200.

9. "Some Mushroom Varieties Sprout More Than Just Good Taste," *Environmental Nutrition* 17 (1994):7.

10. Most of these health benefits can be attributed to a compound in maitake mushrooms called beta 1.6 glucan, a polysaccharide widely recognized as an immune-enhancement compound: A. Cichoke, "Maitake Mushrooms: A Leap Beyond the Ordinary," *Total Health* 16 (1994):20.

11. "Some Mushroom Varieties Sprout More Than Just Good Taste," *Environmental Nutrition* 17 (1994):7; H. Nanba, Kobe Pharmaceutical University, from a paper published by the Pharmaceutical Society of Japan, October, 1994, Kobe, Japan.

12. One study showed that maitake-mushroom extract inhibited breast cancer tumor growth by 70 percent in animals when administered orally, and up to 90 percent when injected directly into the abdominal cavity: F. Murray, "Miraculous Maitake," *Better Nutrition for Today's Living* 57 (1995):50. Other Japanese research has suggested that maitake-mushroom extract exhibits anti-tumor activity against various cancers, probably by activating macrophages to attack tumors and by increasing immune function: H. Nanba, "Anti-tumor Activity of Orally Administered D-fraction from Maitake Mushroom," *Journal of Naturopathic Medicine* 4

(1992):10-15.

13. R. Kennedy, "Mushrooms: They're Not Just for Dinner, They're Culinary Medicine," *Total Health* 17 (1995):27.

14. "Researcher Claims That Mushroom Helps Block HIV," *AIDS Weekly*, March 22, 1993, 4.

15. F. Murray, "Miraculous Maitake," *Better Nutrition for Today's Living* 57 (1995):50.

16. William H. Lee et al., *The Medicinal Benefits of Mushrooms*, New Canaan, Conn.: Keats Publishing, 1985.

17. Shari Lieberman and Nancy Bruning, *The Real Vitamin and Mineral Book*, Garden City Park, N.Y.: Avery Publishing Group, 1990, 352-353.

18. A. Klausner, "Kombucha Tea: Miracle Cure-all or Health Risk?" *Environmental Nutrition* vol. 18, no. 8 (1995): 2.

19. Ginger has been shown to be more effective than Dramamine in preventing motion sickness when taken in a powdered encapsulated form. In one study, a group of college students who were highly susceptible to motion sickness were given either powdered ginger or dimenhydrinate, an anti-nausea meication, and then tested for nausea in rotating chairs. Ginger root was found to be far superior in preventing motion sickness, and other studies have confirmed these results: D. B. Mowrey et al., *Lancet* 1 (1982):655-657.

20. D. B. Mowrey, "Ginger Root: A Blessing for the Gastrointestinal Tract," *Health News & Review*, Spring 1995, 18; Daniel B. Mowrey, *The Scientific Validation of Herbal Medicine*, Cormorant Books, 1986.

21. D. B. Mowrey, "Ginger Root: A Blessing for the Gastrointestinal Tract," *Health News & Review*, Spring 1995, 18.

22. In one study, a group of pregnant women with morning sickness were given either powdered ginger root in capsule form or a placebo. Of those who received the root, 70 percent said they experienced significantly fewer bouts of nausea: W. Fischer-Rasmussen et al., "Ginger Treatment of Hyperemesis Gravidirum," *European Journal of Obstetrics & Gynecology and Reproductive Biology* 38 (1990):1.

23. Paul Schulick, *Common Spice or Wonder Drug? Ginger*, Brattleboro, Vt.: Herbal Free Press, 1993; Daniel B. Mowrey, *The Scientific Validation of Herbal Medicine*, Cormorant Books, 1986; S. Gujral et al., "Effect of Ginger Oleoresin on Serum and Hepatic Cholesterol Levels in Cholesterol Fed Rats," *Nutrition Reports International* 17 (1978):183-189.

24. A water extract of ginger root was found to significantly inhibit platelet aggregation: K. C. Srivastava, "Effects of Aqueous Extracts of Onion, Garlic, and Ginger on Platelet Aggregation and Metabolism of Arachidonic Acid in the Blood Vascular System," *Prostaglandins Leukotrienes and Medicine* 13 (1984):227-235. A number of other studies have comfirmed these results: K. C. Srivastava, "Effect of Onion and Ginger Consumption on Platelet Thromboxane Production in Humans," *Prostaglandins Leukotrienes and Essential Fatty Acids* 35 (1989):183-185; A. I. Kharazi et al., "Platelet Aggregation Inhibiting Drug Containing [6]-Shogaol," *Chemical Abstract* 109 (1988):11.

25. B. K. Khmetova, "The Electrocardiographic Changes in Patients with Chronic

Pulmonary and Pulmonary Cardiac Insufficiency Treated with European Wild Ginger," *Sbornik Nauchnykh Trudov Bashkirskii Meditsinskii Institut* 17 (1968):113-118; T. Kosuge et al., "Isolation and Identification of Cardiac Principles from Laminaria," *Yakugaku Zasshi*, 103 (1983):683–685.

26. Lewis Harrison, *Making Fats and Oils Work for You*, New York: Avery Publishing Group, 1990.

27. James F. Balch, M.D., and Phyllis A. Balch, C.N.C., *Prescription for Nutritional Healing*, New York: Avery Publishing Group, 1990.

28. EPO, BCO, and borage were found to reduce blood pressure in animals, with EPO being the most effective: M. M. Engler, "Comparative Study of Diets Enriched with Evening Primrose, Black Currant, Borage, or Fungal Oils on Blood Pressure and Pressor Responses in Spontaneously Hypertensive Rats," *Prostaglandins Leukotrienes Essential Fatty Acids* 49 (1993):809. In a similar study, borage oil was found to significantly decrease blood pressure in both normal and hypertensive animals and was found to lower systolic blood pressure by as much as 24 percent: M. M. Engler et al., "Dietary GLA Lowers Blood Pressure and Alters Aortic Reactivity and Cholesterol Metabolism in Hypertension," *Journal Hypertension* 10 (1992):1197; M. M. Engler, "Effects of Dietary Borage Oil Rich in GLA on Blood Pressure and Vascular Activity," *Nutrition Research* 12 (1992):519. Blood pressure was also found to be lowered by consumption of GLA concentrate: J. L. Deferne et al., "The Antihypertensive Effect of Dietary Supplementation with a 6-Desaturated EFA Concentrate as Compared with Sunflower Seed Oil," *Journal Human Hypertension* 6 (1992):113. Various other studies have consistently verified these findings.

29. In a one-year human trial, a group of angioplasty patients who were given 270 mg of GLA per day had only a 17 percent occurrence of blockages, while the control group had a 48 percent occurrence: D. F. Horrobin and J. C. Stewart, "Method of Preventing Reocclusion of Arteries," Canadian Patent Application 2,084,273 (December 1, 1992). BCO can inhibit vessel-wall thrombogenicity, a condition that may lead to arterial blockages: M. C. Bertomeu et al., "Selective Effects of Dietary Fats on Vascular 12-HODE Synthesis and Platelet/Vessel Wall Interactions," *Thrombosis Research* 59 (1990):819. Other studies show that EPO supplementation for 30 days (using six capsules of 270 mg of GLA per day) in patients with recent transient ischemic attack—an interruption in blood flow to the brain—reduced the tendency of blood to clot: M. Prencipe et al., "Naudicelle and Platelet Reactivity in TIA Patients," *Italian Journal of Neurologic Sciences* 4 (1982):373.

30. EPO may lower cholesterol levels in both humans and animals: A. K. Dutta-Roy et al., "Effects of Linoleic and Gamma Linoleic Acid on Fatty Acid-Binding Proteins of Rat Liver," *Molecular Cellular Biochemistry* 98 (1990):177. EPO can significantly lower blood triglyceride levels as well, which can further reduce the risk of heart disease: P. Singer et al., "Blood Pressure and Serum Lipids from SHR after Diets Supplemented with Evening Primrose, Sunflower Seed, or Fish Oil," *Prostaglandins Leukotrienes and Essential Fatty Acids* 40 (1990):17. In one study, high levels (1100

and 1600 mg per day) of GLA in the form of EPO were administered to healthy men. The study was designed to provide the same amount of GLA available from the recommended amount of dietary linoleic acid, found in oils, nuts, seeds, whole grains, and eggs. Over one month, researchers found a marked decrease in total cholesterol and LDL cholesterol: J. L. Richard, "Effects of Dietary Intake of GLA on Blood Lipids and Phospholipid Fatty Acids in Healthy Human Subjects," *Journals Clinical Biochemistry and Nutrition* 8 (1990):75. Another study demonstrated that patients who received 3.6 grams a day of EPO for two months showed a significant decrease in overall cholesterol levels and LDL levels: T. Ishikawa et al., "Effects of GLA on Plasma Lipoproteins and Apolipoproteins," *Atherosclerosis* 75 (1989):95.

31. In one study, 9 to 18 grams of EPO were given to a group of patients with malignant tumors. Most of the patients showed significant improvement, including weight gain and tumor reduction: C. F. Van de Merwe et al., "Oral GLA in 21 Patients with Untreatable Malignancy," *British Journal of Clinical Practice* 41 (1987):907. Other studies have confirmed these findings. A number of research reports have noted that GLA can selectively kill cancer cells, and in human studies, most patients have shown substantial response to GLA supplementation or injection: M. R. C. Naidu et al., "Intratumoral GLA Therapy of Human Gliomas," *Prostaglandins Leukotrienes and Essential Fatty Acids* 45 (1992):181.

32. M. E. Begin et al., "Polyunsaturated Fatty Acid Induced Cytotoxicity against Tumor Cells and Its Relationship to Lipid Peroxidation," *Journal of the National Cancer Institute* 80 (1988):188.

33. One study showed that GLA killed cancer cells four times more effectively than DHA: M. E. Begin et al., "Levels of Thiobarbituric Acid Reactive Substances and the Cytocidal Potential of GLA and DHA on ZR-75-1 and CV-1 Cells," *Lipids* 27 (1992):147.

34. C. A. Gonzalez et al., "Borage Consumption as a Possible Gastric Cancer Protective Factor," *Cancer Epidemiology Biomarkers & Prevention* 2 (1993):157.

35. G. Ramesh et al., "Effect of EFAs on Tumor Cells," *Nutrition* 8 (1992):343; S.H.A. El-Ela et al., "Effects of Dietary Primrose Oil on Mammary Tumorigenesis Induced by 7,12 Dimethylbenz(a)anthracene," *Lipids* 22 (1987):1041.

36. H. P. T. Ammon et al., "Pharmacology of *Curcuma longa*," *Planta Medica* 57 (1991): 1-7.

37. J. K. Lin, "Molecular Mechanism of Action of Curcumin," *Journal of the American Chemical Society* (1994): 196–203.

38. A. C. P. Reddy et al., "Studies on Spice Principles as Antioxidants in the Inhibition of Lipid Peroxidation of Rat Liver Microsomes," *Molecular and Cellular Biochemistry* 111 (1992):117.

39. In one study, 500 mg of curcuminoids per day were given to a group of healthy people. After seven days, blood lipid peroxides were 33 percent lower, and blood-cholesterol levels were 29 percent lower: K. B. Soni et al., "Effect of Oral Curcumin Administration on Serum Peroxides and Cholesterol Levels in Human Volun-

teers," *Indian Journal of Physiology and Pharmacology* 36 (1992):273-293.

40. R. Srivastava et al., "Antithrombotic Effect of Curcumin," *Thrombosis Research* 40 (1985):413-417.

41. In one study of patients with oral cancer, some patients showed a dramatic response within only a matter of days. In long-term smokers, curcumin enhances the body's ability to detoxify cigarette-smoke mutagens and carcinogens: K. Usha et al., "The Possible Mode of Action of Cancer Chemopreventive Spice, Turmeric," *Journal of the American College of Nutrition* 13 (1994):519; K. Polasa et al., "Effect of Turmeric on Urinary Mutagens in Smokers," *Mutagenesis* 7 (1992):107. Other phenolic compounds found in turmeric inhibit carcinogenesis and tumor promotion: M. Nagabhusahan et al., "Curcumin as an Inhibitor of Cancer," *Journal of the American College of Nutrition* 11 (1992):192-198; M. T. Huang et al., "Inhibitory Effects of Curcumin on in Vitro Lipoxygenase and Cyclooxygenase Activities in Mouse Epidermis," *Cancer Research* 51 (1991):813-19. Supplementation of 1 percent turmeric in the daily diet inhibited stomach tumors and mammary tumor in animals: M. Nagabhushan et al., "Antimutagenicity and Anticarcinogenicity of Turmeric," *Journal of Nutrition and Cancer* 4 (1987):83 and was shown to reduce the rate of benign and malignant tumor development: M. A. Azuine et al., "Protective Single/Combined Treatment with Betel Leaf and Turmeric Against Methyl Nitrosamine Induced Hamster Oral Carcinogenesis," *International Journal of Cancer* 51 (1992):4653. Curcumin also had a protective effect against skin tumors and colon cancer. In human studies, a dilute ointment applied to skin-cancer lesions reduced itching and pain in more than 50 percent of the patients: R. Kuttan et al., "Turmeric and Curcumin as Topical Agents in Cancer Therapy," *Tumori* 2 (1987):29.

42. Extracts from turmeric and curcuminoids inhibit the growth of bacteria, fungi, and intestinal parasites: H. P. T. Ammon et al., "Pharmacology of *Curcuma longa*," *Planta Medica* 57 (1991):1 and inhibit the production of aflatoxins, produced by the *Aspergillus* mold in contaminated foods: K. B. Soni et al., "Reversal of Aflatoxin Induced Liver Damage by Turmeric and Curcumin," *Cancer Letter* 66 (1992):115.

43. A number of diseases, including rheumatoid arthritis, and external physical traumas, such as injury and surgery, can cause inflammation. Steroids and other anti-inflammatory drugs are generally used to treat inflammation, but can have deleterious side effects, including increases in blood pressure. Turmeric can naturally help treat inflammation, and studies have borne out its efficacy as an anti-inflammatory agent. Oral doses of curcumin in animals were able to reduce tissue swelling by 50 percent: R. C. Srimal et al., "Pharmacology of Diferuloyl Methane (Curcumin), a Non-steroidal Anti-Inflammatory Agent," *Journal of Pharmacy and Pharmacology* 25 (1973):447. In human studies, the anti-inflammatory actions of curcumin were tested on patients who had recently undergone surgery or suffered physical trauma. Researchers found that 400 mg a day of curcumin three times a day for five days resulted in a significant reduction in inflammation and was as effective as treatment with pharmaceutical drugs: R. R. Satoskar et al., "Com-

parison of Anti-Inflammatory Activities of Various Extracts," *Indian Journal of Medical Research* 64 (1986):601. The anti-inflammatory actions of turmeric show great promise in the treatment of arthritis. In one study of patients diagnosed with rheumatoid arthritis, doses of 1200 mg of curcumin a day for five to six weeks led to a significant improvement in all patients, with decreased morning stiffness and increased physical endurance: S. D. Deodhar et al., "Preliminary Studies on Anti-rheumatic Activity of Curcumin," *Indian Journal of Medical Research* 71 (1980):632.

44. C. V. De Wahlly et al., "Flavonoids Inhibit the Oxidative Modification of Low Density Lipoproteins," *Biochemical Pharmacology* 39 (1990):1743-1749; A. Negre-Salvagyre et al., "Quercetin Prevents the Cytotoxicity of Oxidized Low Density Lipoproteins by Macrophages," *Free Radical Biology and Medicine* 12 (1992):101-106.

45. Tea may inhibit the formation and growth of tumors by virtue of its polyphenolic compounds: C. S. Yang et al., "Tea and Cancer," *Journal of the National Cancer Institute* 85 (1993):13, 1038. A study at Rutgers University found that animals who consumed green tea instead of plain drinking water had fewer skin tumors and that green tea substantially decreased the number and size of skin tumors. Overall, the animals had 70 to 90 percent fewer tumors than mice who drank only water: "Green Tea May Have Inhibitory Effect on Skin Tumors," *Cancer Weekly*, March 16, 1992, 3; H. McCord, "More Good News in Tea Leaves," *Prevention* 47 (1995):51. Another study, at the Skin Diseases Research Center at Cleveland's Case Western Research University, found that green tea protects against skin cancer caused by exposure to sunlight. Additionally, benign lumps were not as likely to become cancerous in animals who were given green tea, and topical application of the active compounds in tea reduced adverse reactions to exposure to the sun.

46. "Can Green Tea Offset Some of the Effects of Smoking?" *Nutrition Research Newsletter* 14 (1995):89.

47. "The Greening of Orange Pekoe," *Harvard Health Letter* 19 (1994):8.

48. "Reading Tea Leaves for Health Benefits," *Tufts University Diet & Nutrition Letter* 13 (1995):4.

49. K. Imai et al., "Cross-sectional Study of Effects of Drinking Green Tea on Cardiovascular and Liver Diseases," *British Medical Journal* 310 (1995):693-697.

50. V. M. Parachin, "Foods That Heal and Protect," *Total Health* 17 (1995):14.

51. M. T. Murray, *The Healing Power of Herbs*, Rocklin, Calif.: Prima Publications, 1992, 223-230.

52. The progression of cataracts was halted in 97 percent of patients in a 1989 study that combined bilberry extract and vitamin E. In another study, a remarkable 75 percent of people with nearsightedness showed significant improvement: R. McCaleb, "Bilberry for Circulatory Health," *Better Nutrition for Today's Living* 55 (1993):54. Another study involving patients with diverse eye problems showed that, after consumption of bilberry extract, all experienced relief from their symptoms: A. Scharrer et al., "Anthocyanosides in the Treatment of Retinopathies," *Klinische Monatsblaetter fuer Augenheilkunde* 178 (1981):386-389. Bilberry also increases circulation to the eyes and helps improve the ability to focus—in one 1987

clinical study in Italy, bilberry was shown to improve circulation to the eyes by 80 percent: B. Mars, "Seeing Is Believing the Many Benefits of Bilberry," *Let's Live,* September 1995, 68-69.

53. R. McCaleb, "Bilberry for Circulation," *Better Nutrition for Today's Living* 54 (1992):28.

54. R. McCaleb, "Bilberry for Circulation," *Better Nutrition for Today's Living* 54 (1992):28; R. McCaleb, "Bilberry for Circulatory Health," *Better Nutrition for Today's Living* 55 (1993):54.

55. B. Gruskin, "Chlorophyll—Its Therapeutic Place in Acute and Suppurative Disease," *American Journal of Surgery* 19 (1940):1.

56. J. F. Scheer, "Green is Gold for a Healthful Diet," *Better Nutrition for Today's Living* 57 (1995):52.

57. R. L. Seibold, *Cereal Grass: Nature's Greatest Health Gift,* New Canaan, Conn.: Keats Publishing, 1994.

58. Y. Hagiwara, *Green Barley Essence: The Ideal Fast Food,* New Canaan, Conn.: Keats Publishing, 1986, 1-22.

59. S. Hartman, "Barley Grass: Nature's Own Antacid," *Healthy and Natural Journal* 2 (1995):90-91.

60. B. H. S. Lau et al., "Edible Plant Extracts Modulate Macrophage Activity and Bacterial Mutagenesis," *International Clinical Nutrition Review* 12 (1992):3.

61. J. F. Scheer, "Green Foods," *Better Nutrition for Today's Living* 55 (1993):46; J. F. Scheer, "Green is Gold for a Healthful Diet," *Better Nutrition for Today's Living* 57 (1995):53; "Green Barley Grass May Help Arthritics," *Better Nutrition for Today's Living* 57 (1995):32.

62. J. F. Scheer, "Green is Gold for a Healthful Diet," *Better Nutrition for Today's Living* 57 (1995):54.

63. J. F. Scheer, "Assessing the Buffet of Green Foods," *Better Nutrition for Today's Living* 56 (1994):46.

64. Dr. Chiu Nan Lai of the University of Texas Health Sciences Center in Houston presented a paper at the 1979 meeting of the American Chemical Society suggesting that wheat grass has anti-cancer properties. Research showed that wheat-grass extracts decrease the ability of mutagens to cause cancer by as much as 99 percent. Later studies showed that wheat-grass extract inhibited the cancer-causing effects of benzopyrene and methylcholanthrene: J. F. Scheer, "Green Foods," *Better Nutrition for Today's Living* 55 (1993):46; R. L. Seibold, *Cereal Grass: What's in It for You,* Lawrence, Kans.: Wilderness Community Education Foundation, 1990.

65. R. Conant, "The Greening of the American Diet," *Healthy and Natural Journal* 2 (1995):89; J. F. Scheer, "Green is Gold for a Healthful Diet," *Better Nutrition for Today's Living* 57 (1995):52.

66. "Health Benefits of Spirulina," *HerbalGram* 32 (1994):12.

67. J. F. Scheer, "Assessing the Buffet of Green Foods," *Better Nutrition for Today's Living* 56 (1994):46; Daniel B. Mowrey, *The Scientific Validation of Herbal Medicine,* Cormorant Books, 1986.

68. S. Foster, "Nature's Penicillin," *Mother Earth News* 148 (1995):20; M. Bricklin, *The Practical Encyclopedia of Natural Healing,* Emmaus, Pa.: Rodale Press, 1976, 28-29,

202-203.

69. S. Foster, "Ginkgo: Leaves of Life," *Better Nutrition for Today's Living* 57 (1995):46.

70. F. Murray, *Ginkgo Biloba*, New Canaan, Conn.: Keats Publishing, 1993.

71. M. Bricklin, "Herbs That Turn Back the Clock," *Prevention* 47 (1995):7, 19.

72. M. Bricklin, "Herbs That Turn Back the Clock," *Prevention* 47 (1995):7, 19.

73. In one study, more than 300 patients with cerebral insufficiency—a term that roughly describes a collection of symptoms ranging from memory loss to dizziness to mood disorders—were given 150 mg of ginkgo per day. After three months, 71 percent of the patients treated with ginkgo showed marked improvement: E. Bruchert et al., *Wirksamkeit, Wochenschrift* 133 (1991): S9-S14.

74. J. Kleinjnen et al., *"Ginkgo biloba,"* *Lancet* 340 (1992):1136-1140.

75. D. Mohr et al., "Dietary Supplementation with Coenzyme Q10 Results in Increased Levels of Ubiquinol-10 within Circulating Lipoproteins and Increased Resistance of Human LDL to the Initiation of Lipid Peroxidation," *Biochimica et Biophysica Acta* 1126 (1992):247-254.

76. T. M. Florence, "The Role of Free Radicals in Disease," *Australia New Zealand Journal Ophthalmology* 23 (1995):3-7.

77. James F. Balch, M.D., and Phyllis A. Balch, C.N.C., *Prescription for Nutritional Healing,* New York: Avery Publishing Group, 1990, 10.

78. Jean Carper, *Stop Aging Now!,* New York:HarperCollins, 1995, 138-147.

79. In one large trial in Italy, patients who took 100 to 150 mg of co-Q 10 per day appeared to have fewer heart complications: Y. Hanaki et al., "Coenzyme Q-10 and Coronary Artery Disease," *Clinical Investigator* 71, suppl. 134 (1993): Patients who took 100 mg a day of co-Q 10 for three months showed increased endurance to physical exercise and reported an increased feeling of well being: *Journal of Cardiac Failure* 1 (1995):101. In patients with heart disease, co-Q 10 at 150 mg a day increased exercise performance and reduced acidosis associated with exercise: D. Bendahan et al., "P NMR Spectroscopy and Ergometer Exercise Test as Evidence for Muscle Oxidative Performance Improvements with Coenzyme Q in Mitrochondrial Myopathies," *Neurology* 42 (1992):1203-1208. One eight-year-long study reported that more than 400 patients with heart disease who were treated with co-Q 10 (in doses ranging from 75 to 600 mg per day) showed significant improvement in heart function. Overall, about 87 percent showed substantial improvement, and during the study 43 percent of the patients decreased their medication: H. Jangsjoen, "Usefulness of Coenzyme Q10 in Clinical Cardiology: A Long-term Study," *Molecular Aspects of Medicine,* suppl., 15 (1994): 165-175.

80. K. Lockwood et al., "Progress on Therapy of Breast Cancer with Vitamin Q10 and the Regression of Metastases," *Biochemistry Biophysics Research Communication* 212 (1995):172-177.

81. Patients with various forms of muscular dystrophy were given either a placebo or 100 mg of co-Q 10 in studies conducted at the Institute for Biomedical Research at the University of Texas. Those patients who took co-Q 10 showed a marked improvement in physical health, compared to the placebo patients, who showed no signs of relief. When the placebo group was given co-Q 10, 75 percent of them

showed improvement. The researchers noted that higher levels of co-Q 10, up to 300 to 400 mg per day, would have yielded even greater positive results: K. Folkers et al., "Two Successful Double-Blind Trials with Coenzyme Q-10 (Vitamin Q-10) on Muscular Dystrophy and Neurogenic Atrophies," *Biochimica et Biophysica Acta* 1271 (1995):281-286. In another study, researchers postulated that co-Q 10 can help restore normal function in patients with diabetes-related muscle weakness and relieve excessive weight loss and pain and atrophy in the legs: Y. Suzuki et al., "A Case of Diabetic Amyotrophy Associated with 3243 Mitochondrial RNA Mutation and Successful Therapy with Coenzyme Q10," *Endocrine Journal* 42 (1995):2, 141-145.

BIBLIOGRAPHY AND SUGGESTED READING LIST

Balch, James, M.D., and Phyllis A. Balch. *Prescription for Nutritional Healing.* Garden City Park, NY: Avery Publishing Group, 1990.

Barnard, Neal, M.D. *Food for Life: How the New Four Food Groups Can Save Your Life.* New York: Harmony Books, 1993.

———. *The Power of Your Plate: A Plan for Better Living.* Summertown, TN: Book Publishing Company, 1995.

Berger, Stuart, M.D. *Dr. Berger's Immune Power Diet.* New York: Signet/New American Library, 1985.

Carper, Jean. *Food: Your Miracle Medicine.* New York: Harper Perennial, 1994.

———. *Stop Aging Now! The Ultimate Plan for Staying Young & Reversing the Aging Process.* New York: HarperCollins, 1995.

Clark, Linda. *Know Your Nutrition.* New Canaan, CT: Keats Publishing, 1981.

Erasmus, Udo. *Fats and Oils: The Complete Guide to Fats and Oils in Health and Nutrition.* Vancouver: Alive Publishing, 1986.

Fries, James F., and Lawrence M. Crapo. *Vitality and Aging.* New York: W. H. Freeman and Company, 1981.

Goldberg, Israel, ed. *Functional Foods: Designer Foods, Pharmafoods, Nutraceuticals.* New York: Chapman & Hall, 1994.

Hagiwara, Yoshihide, M.D. *Green Barley Essence.* New Canaan, CT: Keats Publishing, 1985.

Hallowell, Michael. *Herbal Healing: A Practical Introduction to Medicinal Herbs.* Garden City Park, NY: Avery Publishing Group, 1994.

Harrison, Lewis. *Making Fats and Oils Work for You.* Garden City Park, NY: Avery Publishing Group, 1990.

Hausman, Patricia, and Judith Benn Hurley. *The Healing Foods.* Emmaus, PA: Rodale Press, 1989.

Heinerman, John. *The Healing Benefits of Garlic.* New Canaan, CT: Keats Publishing, 1994.

Henrikson, Robert. *Earth Food Spirulina.* Laguna Beach, CA: Ronore Enterprises, 1989.

Hoffman, David. *An Elder's Herbal: Natural Techniques for Promoting Health and Vitality.* Rochester, VT: Healing Arts Press, 1993.

Lin, David J. *Free Radicals and Disease Prevention: What You Must Know.* New Canaan, CT: Keats Publishing, 1993.

Messina, Mark, and Virginia Messina. *The Simple Soybean and Your Health.* Garden City Park, NY: Avery Publishing Group, 1994.

Mowrey, Daniel B. *The Scientific Validation of Herbal Medicine.* Cormorant Books, 1986.

Rath, Matthias, M.D. *Eradicating Heart Disease.* San Francisco: Health Now, 1993.

Salaman, Maureen. *Foods That Heal.* Menlo Park, CA: M.K.S., 1989.

Schulick, Paul. *Common Spice or Wonder Drug?* Brattleboro, VT: Herbal Free Press, 1994.

Seibold, Ronald, ed. *Cereal Grass: Nature's Greatest Health Gift.* New Canaan, CT: Keats Publishing, 1991.

——. *Cereal Grass: What's in It for You!* Lawrence, KS: Wilderness Community Education Foundation, 1990.

Sharma, Hari, M.D. *Freedom from Disease: How to Control Free Radicals.* Toronto: Veda Publishing, 1993.

Tyler, Varro E. *Herbs of Choice: The Therapeutic Use of Phytochemicals.* New York: Pharmaceutical Products Press, 1994.

——. *The Honest Herbal: A Sensible Guide to the Use of Herbs and Related Remedies.* New York: Pharmaceutical Products Press, 1993.

Whitaker, Julian, M.D. *Dr. Whitaker's Guide to Natural Healing.* Rocklin, CA: Prima Publishing, 1995.

Wright, Jonathan, M.D. *Dr. Wright's Guide to Healing with Nutrition.* New Canaan, CT: Keats Publishing, 1990.

INDEX

adrenal function, 63

adzuki (beans). *See* azuki (beans).

AIDS, 62–64, 78

alcohol, 22, 61
  and food poisoning, 61

alcoholism, 67

alfalfa, 74–75

allicin, 58

allium, 57

allylic sulfides, 9, 40, 190
    See also sulfer compounds.

Almada, Anthony, xi, 9, 21, 22, 34

almonds, 33, 35, 52
  and cholesterol, 54
  fat makeup of, 53

alpha-carotene, 9, 18–19, 21, 40, 143, 152
  diseases affected by, 22, 48. *See also* carotenoids.

alpha-linolenic acid, 52

Alzheimer's disease, 14
  and co-Q 10, 35
  and *Ginkgo biloba*, 75

and vitamin E, 35, 54

amaranth, 44
  cooking time, 85

American Diabetes Association, 44

American Heart Association (AHA), 28, 30–31

American Journal of Clinical Nutrition, 54

anasazi (beans), 55
  cooking time, 84

anchovies, 51

anemia, 73

angina, 78

anthocyanins, 60, 71

antioxidants (vitamins), xi, 2, 6, 8, 9, 15, 17, 18, 24, 37–38, 50, 82
  and alfalfa, 74
  and bilberry, 71
  and cancer, 2, 25–27, 46
  and cardiovascular disease, 28
  cereal grasses, 72
  and co-Q 10, 77
  and fruits, 48

and green tea, 69
  and immunity, 32
  major types of, 36–37
  new antioxidants, 59–79
  and nuts, 54
  and whole grains, 43

apricots, 8, 33, 48

arachidoni acid, 66

arthritis, 14, 42
  and barley grass, 73
  and bilberry, 71
  and gamma linolenic acid, 65, 67
  and ginger, 65
  and turmeric, 67

arugula, 47

asbestos, 25

ascorbic acid. *See* vitamin C.

asparagus, 18, 37
  and immunity, 33

Aspergillus, 64

asthma, 63
  and barley grass, 73
  and co-Q 10, 77
  and gamma linolenic acid, 65

and ginger, 65
and *Ginkgo biloba*, 75
astragalus, 29
and immunity, 33
atherosclerosis, 28, 29, 47, 51
and bilberry, 71
and co-Q 10, 77, 78
and garlic, 57
and *Ginkgo biloba*, 75
and mushrooms, 63
and vitamin E, 54
and wine (red), 60
avocados, 18, 33
Tuna Salad Niçoise with Avocado, 162
azuki (beans), 55
cooking time, 84

B vitamins, 2, 16, 35, 44, 45
and beriberi, 1, 16
toxicity, 20
Balch, James, 49
Balch, Phyllis, 49
barley, 33, 43, 44
cooking time, 85
grass, 73
juice, 73
bass (striped), 51
beans, 33, 35, 40, 49, 54–57, 179–189
Azuki Beans and Greens, 189
Baked Chickpea Loaf, 187
Basil–Lentil Stew, 181
canned, 83
Curried Mung Beans, 188
and gas, 8
Garlic Hummus with Roasted Red Peppers, 192
Hot and Spicy Hummus, 186
Lentil–Garlic Paté, 183
Mexican Bean Salad, 182
phytochemicals in, 179
preparation of, 83–84

Simon-and-Garfunkel Black Bean Soup, 184
Three-Bean Indian Dal, 180
Tomato–Bean Salad with Parsley, 88
types of, 55
White Bean Soup with Sage, 185
bee pollen, 34
Beecher, G. R., 19
beets, 33
greens, 18, 47
beriberi, 1, 13, 43
and thiamin, 12
beta-carotene, 9, 14, 15, 17, 18–19, 20, 21, 38, 40, 49, 143, 152
and alfalfa, 74
and barley grass, 73
and cancer, 24–26
and cereal grasses, 72
and co-Q 10, 78
diseases affected by, 22
and greens, 47, 134
and immunity, 32, 33
and spirulina, 74
and T-cells, 32
See also carotenoids.
beta-glucan, 62
bilberry, 29, 70–72
bilobalides, 75
bioflavonoid, 69
biotin, 38
birth defects, 20
bisdemethoxycurcumin, 67
black currants, 33, 36
oil (BCO), 65, 66
black turtle (beans), 55, 56
cooking time, 84
black-eyed peas, 55
cooking time, 84
bladder (the), 48
Block, Gladys, 25
blood, 23, 58
cells (white), 32
clotting, 1, 9, 20, 29, 36

and alfalfa, 74
and gamma linolenic acid, 65
and garlic, 57
and *Ginkgo biloba*, 75
and omega-3 fatty acids, 50, 51
platelets, 69
blood pressure, 1, 23
and alcohol, 61
and alfalfa, 74
and almonds, 54
and barley grass, 73
and bilberry, 71
and chlorella, 74
and co-Q 10, 77
and EFAs, 53
and gamma linolenic acid, 65
and garlic, 58
and green tea, 69
and macadamia nuts, 54
and mushrooms, 62–63
and omega-3 fatty acids, 50
and selenium, 54
See also hypertension.
bluefin, 51
Blumberg, Jeffrey, 32
bok choy, 41
bones, 1, 36
borage, 65–67
boron, 35
Bradlow, H. Leon, 41
Brazil nuts, 33, 52, 54
brewer's yeast, 38
British Journal of Clinical Pharmacology, 76
broccoflower, 41
broccoli, 1, 10, 15, 18, 26, 29, 37, 41
Broccoli–Cauliflower Bisque, 100
Broccoli and Pine Nut Casserole, 96
Broccoli Rabe Stir-Fry, 102
and cancer, 41

and immunity, 33
bronchial constriction, 75
brussels sprouts, 10, 18, 26, 36, 41
  Brussels Sprouts with Honey–Ginger Glaze, 98
buckwheat, 44
  cooking time, 85
bulgur wheat. *See* wheat, bulgur.
butter, 36

cabbage, 10, 18, 36, 37, 41
  and cancer, 41
  and immunity, 33
  Peppered Cabbage Stew, 103
  Red and Green Cabbage Salad, 100
  Wild Mushroom Cabbage Rolls, 101
calcium, 1, 44, 45
  and beans, 55
  and osteoporosis, 2
Camellia sinensis, 68
Cancer Research Center, 40
cancer, 1, 9, 17, 23, 24–27, 41, 43, 51
  and antioxidants, 46
  and beans, 56
  and bilberry, 71
  bladder, 22, 25, 49
  breast, 10, 27, 41, 42, 43, 49, 50, 51, 54, 56, 57, 69, 78
  and caloric restriction, 30
  and carotenoids, 48, 50
  cells, 22, 25, 27
  cervical, 26, 27, 41, 49, 54
  colon, 22, 25, 41, 42, 43, 49, 54, 56, 57, 69
  and co-Q 10, 77, 78
  and dietary fats, 2
  and ellagic acid, 49
  esophagal, 27, 42, 54, 69–70

and fiber, 46, 58
and flavonoids, 49
and garlic, 57
gastrointestinal, 58
and *Ginkgo biloba*, 75
and green tea, 69
increases in rates of, 24
intestinal, 56
and legumes, 55
leukemia, 42, 58
and lignins, 54
and limonoids, 46
liver, 69
lung, 15, 22, 25, 40, 42, 47, 49, 54
mouth, 42, 54
and mushrooms, 62–64
and obesity, 30
and omega-3 fatty acids, 51, 54
and onions, 58
ovarian, 41
pancreatic, 41, 56, 69
prevention of through nutrition, 25–27
prostate, 22, 25, 42, 56
rectal, 43
and selenium, 54
skin, 22, 25, 42, 49
and soybeans, 42
and spinach, 47
and spirulina, 74
stomach, 25, 26, 27, 54, 57
and sulforaphane, 41
throat, 54
and tomatoes, 40
and turmeric, 67
and vegetables, 58
and vitamin A, 50
and vitamin C, 50
and vitamin E, 50
candida, 48, 78
canola oil, 53
cantaloupe, 18, 33, 35, 48
  Cantaloupe Wedges with Frosted Champagne Grapes, 149

canthaxanthin, 22, 40, 63, 143, 153
capillary integrity, 71
carbohydrates, 22
cardiovascular disease, 14, 23, 27–29
  and alcohol, 61
  and barley grass, 73
  and beta-carotene, 28
  and catechins, 29
  and co-Q 10, 77
  and dietary fats, 2
  and fiber, 2
  and flavonoids, 49
  and *Ginkgo biloba*, 75
  and green tea, 69
  and legumes, 55
  and obesity, 30
  and omega-3 fatty acids, 50
  and spirulina, 74
  and turmeric, 67
  and vitamin C, 29
  and vitamin E, 28, 43
  and whole grains, 43
  and wine (red), 60
carotenoids, 8–9, 18–22, 40, 63
  and cancer, 25–26, 48
  and cognitive functions, 35
  diseases affected by, 22, 49
  and fruits, 48–49, 143
  and greens, 47, 134
  and red/orange/yellow vegetables, 49, 152
  sources of, 18–19, 199
  and spirulina, 74
  and tomatoes, 40, 86
  types of, 9
  See also vitamin A.
Carper, J., 35
carrots, 8, 15, 18, 20, 21, 25, 49
  and immunity, 33
Cartier, Jacques, 47
cashews, 52

cataracts, 41, 46
  and carotenoids, 49
catechins, 60
cauliflower, 33, 41
  Broccoli–Cauliflower
    Bisque, 100
  Cauliflower Paratha, 99
cavities, 69, 70
celery, 18, 23
  and immunity, 33
cellulose, 49
cherries, acerola, 33
chestnuts, 52
chickpeas. *See* garbanzo
    (beans).
chicory, 18
chives, 33, 58
chlorella growth factor
    (CGF), 74
chlorella, 73–74
chlorogenic acid, 40, 41, 86
chlorophyll, 72–75
cholesterol, 1, 15, 29, 30, 40
  and beans, 55
  and chlorella, 74
  and co-Q 10, 77
  and EFAs, 53
  and fiber, 46, 48–49
  and fish, 51
  and garlic, 57–58
  and ginger, 65
  and grapefruit, 46
  and grapes, 60
  and green tea, 69
  HDL, 29, 30, 42, 51, 57,
    58, 60, 70, 74
  LDL, 28, 29, 42, 43, 51,
    54, 55, 57, 58, 60, 66,
    69, 70, 78
  and legumes, 55
  and nuts, 52–54
  and obesity, 30
  and onions, 58
  and resveratrol, 60–61
  and seeds, 52
  and soybeans, 42
  and spinach, 47

  and spirulina, 74
  and turmeric, 67
  VLDL, 50
  and whole grains, 43
chromium, 29
cigarettes (smoking), 25, 31
  and hypertension, 31
  and green tea, 69–70
cilantro
  Cilantro Salsa, 94
  Cilantro–Walnut Tabouli,
    121
  Cilantro–Walnut Tofu, 110
citrus fruits. *See* fruits,
    citrus.
co-Q 10 (coenzyme Q10),
    7, 9, 29, 77–79. *See also*
    isoprenoids.
  and Alzheimer's disease, 35
  and immunity, 33
coconut
  Coconut-Curried udon,
    116
  Carrot–Coconut Bisque,
    155
cod, 24, 29
cod-liver oil, 33
Colditz, Graham, 40
colitis, 49
collard greens, 18, 41, 47
constipation, 49, 62, 73
*Consumed: Why Americans
    Love, Hate, and Fear
    Food,* 12
copper, 38
corn, 18, 43, 44
  grits, 85
  and immunity, 33
  oil, 77
coumarin, 40, 190
couscous, 44
  cooking time, 85
cranberries, 48
creatine, 34
cryptoxanthin, 18–19, 40,
    48, 143, 152. *See also*
    carotenoids.

curcumin, 67–68
curry
  Coconut-Curried Udon, 116
  Curried Greens, 135
  Curried Mung Beans, 188
  Curried Yam Soup, 159
  Indian Vegetable Curry, 97
cyanohydroxybutene
    (CHB), 41

D-limonene, 9, 46. *See also*
    limonoids; terpenoids.
dandelion greens, 33, 47
Decision Resources
    (consulting firm), 7
DeFelice, Stephen L., xi,
    12, 15
demethoxycurcumin, 67
designer foods, 6
  definition of, 7
diabetes, 14, 42
  and barley grass, 73
  and co-Q 10, 77
  and fiber, 43, 49, 56
  and gamma linolenic acid,
    65, 67
  and mushrooms, 62–63
  and spirulina, 74
diallyl disulfide (DADS), 57
dietary fats, 2
dill, 18
docosahexaenoic acid
    (DHA), 50–51, 52
Dreamy Orange-Cream
    Freeze, 129
Duke, James, 54
dysentery, 57

eczema, 67
eggs, 36, 38
eicosapentaenoic acid
    (EPA), 50–51, 52
elderberries, 33
ellagic acid, 40, 143, 170, 190
  and cancer, 54, 58
  and red/orange/yellow
    vegetables, 49, 152

Elmer, Gary, 35, 47
endive, 18, 33, 47
epigallocatechin gallate
    (EGCG), 69
epsilon-carotene, 9
Escherichia (E.) coli, 61
essential fatty acids (EFAs),
    9, 52–54, 66
    sources of, 200
    types of, 9

fava beans, 84
fennel, 18
    Fennel with Red Onions,
        198
fenugreek, 23
fever, 14
fettucccini
    Whole-Wheat Fettuccini
        with Salmon and Sage,
        124
fiber, 2, 6, 15, 22, 40, 44
    and beans, 55–56, 179
    and cancer, 27, 43, 46, 58
    and cardiovascular
        disease, 2
    and cholesterol, 46
    and cruciferous veg-
        etables, 40, 41, 95
    and diabetes, 43
    and fruits, 48, 143
    and red/orange/yellow
        vegetables, 49, 152
    types of, 9, 46, 49
    and whole grains, 43, 114
filberts, 52
Find/SVP, 17
First International Gastric
    Cancer Congress, 47
fish, 40, 50–51
    Grilled Mako with
        Orange Pepper
        Champagne Glaze, 169
    Grilled Swordfish with
        Snow Peas and Water
        Chestnuts, 164
    Hearty Fish Chowder, 163

oil(s), 23, 36, 50–51, 66
    recipes, 160–169
    Salmon Paté with Roasted
        Red Pepper and
        Chives, 161
    Salmon-Stuffed Mush-
        rooms, 165
    San Francisco Cioppino,
        87
    Seafood Etouffée, 167
    Sesame–Ginger Shrimp,
        176
    Smoked Salmon Salad
        with Lemon–Honey
        Cucumbers, 168
    Tuna–Olive Paté, 169
    Tuna Salad Niçoise with
        Avocado, 162
    and vitamin E, 51
    White Peppercorn Mako
        with Capers, 166
    Whole-Wheat Fettuccini
        with Salmon and Sage,
        124
    zoochemicals in, 160
flatulence, 67
flavonoids, 9, 29, 39, 40,
    190
    and bilberry, 71
    and cancer, 49, 58
    and *Ginkgo biloba,* 75
    and nuts, 54
    types of, 9
    and wine (red), 60
flaxseed oil, 27, 53, 54
    and lignins, 54
    and omega-3 fatty acids,
        54
folic acid, 35, 38, 40, 175
    and cancer, 41, 47
    and cruciferous veg-
        etables, 95
    and greens, 47, 134
    and heart disease, 47
Food and Drug Administra-
    tion, The (FDA), 15, 61
Food: Your Miracle Medicine, 35

Forman, M. R., 19
Forsyth Dental Center, 70
Foundation for Innovation
    in Medicine, xi
free radicals, 21, 25, 29, 35–
    38
    and cell damage, 37
    and co-Q 10, 77
    and enzymes, 37
    and exercise, 34–35
    and green tea, 69
    and hypertension, 31
    and immunity, 32
    and soybeans, 42
    and turmeric, 67
fruits, 17, 25, 26, 27, 35, 40,
    60
    citrus, 9, 29, 40, 45–46
        Asparagus with Ginger-
            Orange Glaze, 128
        Blood Orange Ambro-
            sia, 131
        and cataracts, 46
        Citrus Salad with Spiced
            Raisins and Jicama,
            126
        and fiber, 49
        Grapefruit and Kiwi
            Salad on Field Greens,
            127
        Honeydew Lime Cooler,
            129
        Iced Berry Lemonade,
            127
        and immunity, 33
        Lemonberry Muffins,
            133
        and phytochemicals, 125
        Skinny Lemon Caper
            Sauce, 130
        Tangerine Dream, 132
    and ellagic acid, 54
    and fiber, 49
    red/orange/yellow, 48–49
        Cantaloupe Wedges with
            Frosted Champagne
            Grapes, 149

Mango–Banana Freeze, 150
Mango–Raisin Salsa, 150
Mixed Greens with Mango Glaze, 147
and phytochemicals, 143
Raspberry–Pecan Crunch, 146
Red Grapefruit Ambrosia, 148
Strawberry Dream Pie, 151
Vanilla–Berry Butter, 174
Veronica's Very Special Apricot Peach Tart, 145
Very Berry Sauce, 144
Watermelon Slushie, 144
Super Berry Smoothie
Thelma's Raspberry Sort-Of Cheesecake, 113
functional foods, 1, 2, 6, 27
definition of, 7
See also nutraceuticals.
Functional Foods: Designer Foods, Pharmafoods, Nutraceuticals, 32

gallbladder diseases, 30
gamma linolenic acid (GLA), 65–67. *See also* black currant, oil (BCO); borage; omega-6 essential fatty acid; primrose oil (EPO).
garbanzo (beans), 55, 56
cooking time, 84
garlic, 1, 9, 14, 23, 40
and cardiovascular disease, 29
extract, 13
and cancer, 27, 39
and immunity, 33
and onions, 57–58
Baked Garlic Cloves, 197
Creamy Garlic Sauce, 193
Fennel with Red Onions, 198

French Onion Soup, 195
Garlic-Baked Jalapeno Bites, 194
Garlic Hummus with Roasted Red Peppers, 192
Garlic-Stuffed Red Peppers, 191
Garlic–Toasted Nut Mix, 108
Parsley–Garlic Pitas, 197
and phytochemicals, 190
Tarragon–Leek Soup, 196
Tempeh with Garlic Sauce, 109
Wild Mushroom Sauté with Leeks, 198
gastrointestinal disorders, 13
genistein, 10, 40, 104
and cancer, 42
ginger, 14, 64–65
Ginkgo biloba, 29, 35, 75–77
ginkgolic acid, 75
ginkgolides, 75
ginnol, 75
ginseng, 29,
and immunity, 33
Siberian, 34
ginsenin, 33
glaucoma, 71
glutamic acid, 62
glutathione, 40
and citrus fruit, 46, 125
and tomatoes, 41, 86
glycyrrhizin, 27
Goldberg, Israel, 32
Goodman, Michael, 7
grains, whole, 27, 37, 38, 43–45, 49
Almond Rice with Green Peas, 177
Cilantro–Walnut Tabouli, 121
Coconut–Curried Udon, 116
Fragrant Spiced Basmati Rice, 122

and immunity, 33
Lemonberry Muffins, 133
Millet and Summer Squash Casserole, 119
Parsley–Garlic Pitas, 197
Peanut Soba Noodles, 175
Sesame–Herb Bread, 172
Sesame Soba Salad, 115
Seven-Vegetable Pasta with Tarragon Glaze, 117
Spicy Pepper Pasta, 120
Spinach–Mushroom Samosas, 137
Stuffed Red Peppers with Basil-Basmati Rice, 158
types of, 44–45
Walnut–Oat Bread, 123
Whole-Wheat Fettuccini with Salmon and Sage, 124
Wild Rice Salad with Toasted Pecans, 118
grapefruit, 9, 23, 36, 46
and cholesterol, 46
and immunity, 33
pink, 18
red, 48
grapes, 49
Cantaloupe Wedges with Frosted Champagne Grapes, 149
juice, 60–61
red, 48
Great Northern beans, 84
greens, 46–47
Azuki Beans and Greens, 189
Baked Kale with Parsnips and Carrots, 141
Beets and Field Greens with Walnuts, 157
Braised Swiss Chard, 138
Collard and Carrot Raita, 138
Creamy Spinach Sage Soup, 136

Curried Greens, 135
Double Delicious Pesto, 177
Grapefruit and Kiwi Salad on Field Greens, 127
Mixed Greens with Mango Glaze, 147
Mixed Greens Stew, 140
Palak Paneer, 139
and phytochemicals, 134
Southern Style Turnip Greens, 139
Spicy Gingered Greens, 142
Spinach–Mushroom Samosas, 137
Sunny Sprouted Avocado Salad, 173
guava, 33, 36, 49
  juice, 18
gum disease, 69, 70
gum(s), 49

headaches, 65
  and *Ginkgo biloba*, 75, 76, 77
heart disease, 2, 13, 21, 24, 30, 43, 47, 49, 54. *See also* cardiovascular disease.
hemicellulose, 49
hemorrhoids, 49
  and mushrooms, 63
Hennekens, Charles, 25
herbs, 2
herring, 33
Hippocrates Health Institute, 73
hippuric acid, 48
Holden, J. M., 19
homocysteine, 47
horseradish, 33
human immunodeficiency virus (HIV), 62–63
  and sulfolipids, 74
hydrazines, 62
hydrogen peroxide, 37
hydroxyl radical, 37

hypertension, 14, 23, 29–31
  and cigarette smoking, 31
  and obesity, 31
  and sodium, 2
  and stroke, 30

immunity, 2, 13, 22, 23, 31–33
  and chlorella, 74
  and co-Q 10, 77, 78
  enhancers, 33
  and fish oils, 51
  and garlic, 33
  and mushrooms, 63
  recipes. *See* Basil–Lentil Stew; Garlic Hummus; Lentil–Garlic Paté; Roasted Red Peppers; Smoky Shiitake–Brussels Sprouts Salad.
  and selenium, 54
  and whole grains, 43
  and zinc, 2
impotence, 76
indoles, 1, 10, 39, 40, 95
  and cancer, 41
  sources of, 200
  types of, 9
interleukin-1, 62
intermittent claudication, 76
iron, 35, 42, 43, 44, 45
  and beans, 55
isoflavones, 40, 42, 170
  and beans, 56, 179
  and nuts, 54
  and soybeans, 104
isoprenoids, 9
  sources of, 200
  types of, 9
isothiocyanates, 9, 40, 95
  and cancer, 27

Japanese Ministry of Health and Welfare, 7
Journal of the American Dietetic Association, 19
Journal of the American Medical Association, 50

Journal of the National Cancer Institute, 19

kale, 18, 41, 47
kamut, 44
Kaposi sarcoma, 63
Khachik, F., 19
kidney beans, 55, 56
  cooking time, 84
kidney disease, 13, 63, 73
kidneys (human), 48, 74
kiwi, 18
Kleinjnen, Jos, 76
Knipschild, Paul, 76
Kohlmeier, Lenore, 21, 29
Krebs, Ernst, Jr., 73
kumquats, 33

L-carnitine, 34
LaChance, Paul, 38, 39
laetrile, 73
Lanza, E., 19
lectins, 48
leeks, 9, 19, 57, 58
legumes, 35, 38, 40
  and cancer, 55
  and cholesterol, 55
  and gas, 83
  and heart disease, 54–55
  and obesity, 55
  preparation of 83–84
lemons, 9, 45, 46
  and immunity, 33
lenitan, 62
lentils, 55
  cooking time, 84
lentinan, 33
licorice extract, 13
licorice root, 27
life span, 24
lignins, 27, 40, 49, 54, 56, 170
lima beans, 55, 56
  cooking time, 84
limes, 9, 45
  and immunity, 33
limonoids, 9, 40, 46, 125
  and cancer, 46

linoleic acid, 52, 65
linseed oils, 52
lipid peroxidation, 68
lipid peroxy radical
liver (food), 33, 35
liver (human organ), 32, 35, 63, 64, 65, 74
loganberries, 33
lung disease, 9
lutein, 18–19, 40, 134, 143, 152
  diseases affected by, 22, 48
  See also carotenoids.
lycopene, 18–19, 19–20, 21, 40, 143, 152
  diseases affected by, 22, 48
  and tomatoes, 40
  See also carotenoids.
lysine, 45

macadamia nuts, 52, 54
mackeral, 33, 35, 51, 77
macronutrients, 7
macrophages, 32
  and mushrooms, 62
  and spirulina, 74
macular degeneration, 22
  and bilberry, 71
  and carotenoids, 49
  and spinach, 47
manganese, 33, 38
Mangles, R. A., 19
mangos, 19, 36, 48
  and immunity, 33
Marcozzi, M. S., 19
meats
  organ, 36. *See also* liver (food).
  red, 35
melanoma, 27
menstruation, 53
microbiotics, 12
micronutrients, 7
milk, 35
millet, 33, 44
  cooking time, 85

Millet and Summer Squash Casserole,119
mitochondria, 34, 77
molasses (blackstrap), 33
monoterpenes, 9
Morris, Dexter, 19–21, 28–29
motorneuron disease, 14
mucilages, 49
multiple sclerosis, 67
mung beans, 55
  cooking time, 84
muscular dystrophy, 78
musculoskeletal system, 74
mushrooms, 33, 61–64
  button, 83
  Hot Gingered Tomatoes, 94
  kombucha, 63–64
  maitake, 62
  medicinal, 29
  Nice and Nutty Veggie Burgers, 178
  reishi, 63
  Salmon-Stuffed Mushrooms, 165
  shiitake, 33, 62
  Smoky Shiitake–Brussels Sprouts Salad, 98
  Spinach–Mushroom Samosas, 137
  substitutions (in recipes), 83
  Tempeh with Pine Nuts and Morels, 112
  Wild Mushroom Cabbage Rolls, 101
  Wild Mushroom Calzones, 92
  Wild Mushroom Sauté with Leeks, 198
mustard, 9
mustard greens, 18, 41, 47
  and immunity, 33
myocardial infarctions, 29
Myogenix, xi, 9

myrtillin, 71

National Cancer Institute (NCI), 9, 13, 18, 24, 44, 46, 58, 63
nausea, 14, 71, 76
navy beans, 55, 56
  cooking time, 84
nearsightedness, 71
nectarines, 19, 33
neurological degeneration, 14
New England Journal of Medicine, 53
Newsweek, 2
niacin. *See* vitamin B$_3$.
night blindness, 71
nitrosamines, 25, 26
  and garlic, 57
  green tea, 69
  and tomatoes, 41
nutraceuticals, 1, 6, 15
  definition of, 6–7
  See also functional foods.
nutriceuticals. *See* nutraceuticals.
nuts, 28, 33, 35, 37, 40, 49, 52–54, 77
  and seeds, 52–54
  Almond Rice with Green Peas, 177
  Beets and Field Greens with Walnuts, 157
  Broccoli and Pine-Nut Casserole, 96
  Cilantro–Walnut Tabouli, 121
  Cilantro–Walnut Tofu, 110
  Cumin-Roasted Walnuts, 171
  Double Delicious Pesto, 177
  Easy Almond Milk, 174
  Garlic–Toasted Nut Mix, 108
  Nice And Nutty Veggie Burgers, 178

Peanut Soba Noodles, 175
Raspberry–Pecan Crunch,
 146
Sesame–Ginger Shrimp, 176
Sesame–Herb Bread, 172
Sunny Sprouted Avocado
 Salad, 173
Tempeh with Pine Nuts
 and Morels, 112
Vanilla–Berry Butter, 174
Walnut–Oat Bread, 123
Wild Rice Salad with
 Toasted Pecans, 118
 phytochemicals in, 170

oats, 33, 43, 44
 cooking time, 85
obesity, 13, 23, 29–30
 and alfalfa, 74
 and barley grass, 73
 and cancer, 30
 and co-Q 10, 77
 and gamma linolenic acid,
  65
 and spirulina, 74
 and turmeric, 67
 and whole grains, 43
octacosanol, 34
Odyssey Nutriceutical
 Sciences, 14, 24
okra, 19
olive oil, 23
 and immunity, 33
omega-3 (fatty acids), 23,
 29, 40, 50–51, 160
 and cancer, 51
 and flaxseed, 53
omega-6 (fatty acids), 50–
 51, 65–67
onions, 9, 23, 40, 60
 and garlic, 57–58
  Baked Garlic Cloves, 197
  Creamy Garlic Sauce, 193
  Fennel with Red Onions,
   198
  French Onion Soup, 195

Garlic-Baked Jalapeno
  Bites, 194
Garlic Hummus with
  Roasted Red Peppers,
  192
Garlic-Stuffed Red
  Peppers, 191
Garlic–Toasted Nut
  Mix, 108
Lentil–Garlic Paté, 183
Parsley–Garlic Pitas, 197
and phytochemicals, 190
Tarragon–Leek Soup, 196
Wild Mushroom Sauté
  with Leeks, 198
 green, 3
 and immunity, 33
oranges, 9, 26, 36, 46
 and immunity, 33
organic acids, 9
 types of, 9
 sources of, 200
organosulfur, 1, 40, 57, 190
 types of, 9
orthomolecular compo-
  nents, 7
Osband, Michael, 13, 24
osteoporosis, 2
 and calcium, 2
Oxford University, 56
oxidants, 37
oxygen, 37
oysters, 51

p-coumaric acid, 40, 41, 86
Packer, Lester, 34
panaquilon, 33
panaxin, 33
pancreatitis, 73
panoxic, 33
pantothenic acid. See
  vitamin B$_5$.
papayas, 33, 48
parsley, 19, 33, 36, 47
 Tomato–Bean Salad with
  Parsley, 88

Parsley–Garlic Pitas, 197
pasta. See grains.
Pasteur, Louis, 57
Pauling, Linus, 26–27,
 32–33
peaches, 19, 48, 49
peanut(s), 33
 oil, 37
 fat makeup of, 53
peas, 19, 35
 dried, 49
 cooking time, 84
 Grilled Swordfish with
  Snow Peas and Water
  Chestnuts, 164
pectin, 46, 48, 49
pellegra, 43
peppers, bell, 19, 26, 29, 36,
 49
 and immunity, 33
 Salmon Paté with Roasted
  Red Pepper and
  Chives, 161
peridontal disease, 78
persimmons, 33, 36
phenols, 9, 40, 43, 143, 143,
 170
 and cancer, 27, 49
 and red/orange/yellow
  vegetables, 49, 152
 sources of, 199
 and turmeric, 67
 types of, 9
 and whole grains, 43, 114
 and wine (red), 60
phosphorous, 45
 and beans, 55
phycocyanin, 74
phytate, 40, 42, 43, 179
 and beans, 56
 foods rich in, 43
phytic acid, 27, 40, 104, 114
phytochemicals, x–xii, 1, 2,
 8, 15, 39–58, 82
 and beans, 179
 and cancer, 25, 27

categories of, 9
and citrus fruits, 125
and cruciferous vegetables, 95
definition of, 7
and grains, 114
and green tea, 69
and greens, 134
and immunity, 32
and nuts and seeds, 54, 170
and onions and garlic, 190
and red/orange/yellow fruits, 143
and red/orange/yellow vegetables, 49, 152
and soybeans, 104
and tomatoes, 86
phytoestrogens, 40
and soybeans, 42, 104
phytonutrients, 7. *See also* phytochemicals.
Pierson, Herbert, 46
pimentos, 3
pine nuts, 52
recipe, 96
pineapple, 33
pinto beans, 55, 56
cooking time, 84
pistachios, 33, 35, 52
plums, 19
polychlorinated biphenyls (PCBs), 25
and chlorella, 74
polyphenols, 60, 69
polysaccharides, 62
potassium, 55
potatoes, sweet, 19, 49
and immunity, 33
premenstrual syndrome, 66, 67
Prescription for Nutritional Healing, 49
Preventive Nutrition Consultants, 46
primrose oil (EPO), 65–67

proanthocyanidins, 75
prostaglandins (PGs), 66
prostate gland, 54, 74
protease inhibitors, 1, 27, 40, 42, 104
protein, 22, 44
protooncogenes, 25
psyllium, 27
pumpkins, 19, 49
and immunity, 33
seeds, 52
and the prostate gland, 54

quercetin, 40, 58, 75, 190
quinoa, 44–45
cooking time, 85

radicchio
Sautéed Peppers on Braised Radicchio, 157
radishes, 9
and immunity, 33
rapeseed, 52
raspberries, 33, 48, 49
red beans, 84
resveratrol, 60–61
retinol. *See* retinoids; vitamin A.
retinoids, 9
sources of, 200
See also vitamin A.
rheumatoid arthritis, 51
riboflavin. *See* vitamin B$_2$.
rice, 33
cooking times, 85
Spanish Paella, 93
types of, 45
Wild Rice Salad with Toasted Pecans, 118
rickets, 13
Romaine lettuce, 19
Romano, Joseph, 35, 47
rutabagas, 41
Rutgers University, 38, 39
rye, 45

S-allyl-cysteine (SAC), 57
saccharin, 25
safflower, 37, 53
salmon, 24, 29, 51, 77
Salmon Paté with Roasted Red Pepper and Chives, 161
Salmon-Stuffed Mushrooms, 165
Smoked Salmon Salad with Lemon–Honey Cucumbers, 168
Whole-Wheat Fettuccini with Salmon and Sage, 124
salmonella, 61
sardines, 24, 35, 51, 77
and immunity, 33
scallions, 9, 19, 57, 58
Schnabel, Charles, 72
Schweitzer, Albert, 57
Science, 13
scurvy, 1, 12, 16, 45
seafood, 33, 35, 50
selenium, 31, 32, 33, 38
and Brazil nuts, 54
senile dementia, 78
sesame seeds, 33, 35, 37, 52
fat makeup of, 53
Sesame Soba Salad, 115
shallots, 57, 58
shellfish, 35
Silverman, Harold, 35, 47
singlet oxygen, 37
Snowden, David, 40
soy milk, 10, 42, 83
soybean(s), 1, 10, 35, 38, 40, 42–43, 43, 55
Burritos Grande, 106
and cancer, 27
Cilantro–Walnut Tofu, 110
cooking time, 84
Garlic–Toasted Nut Mix, 108
and immunity, 33

meal, 13
oil, 37
phytochemicals in, 104
Red Pepper Tempeh, 107
Spicy Tofu Dal, 105
Spicy Tofu Steaks, 111
Super Berry Smoothie,
    110
Tempeh with Garlic
    Sauce, 109
Tempeh with Pine Nuts
    and Morels, 112
Thelma's Raspberry Sort-
    Of Cheesecake, 113
spelt, 45
Spicy Stuffed Tomatoes, 91
spinach, 19, 36, 37, 47
    and immunity, 33, 47
spirulina, 34, 74
split peas, 55
squash, 19, 33, 36, 49
    and immunity, 33
    summer, 19
    winter, 19
squid, 51
Stacey, Michelle, 12
staphylococcus, 61
Stop Aging Now!, 35
Strang Cornell Cancer
    Research Center, 41
strawberries, 25, 36, 48, 49
    and immunity, 33
stroke, 14
    and alcohol, 61
    and hypertension, 30
    and macadamia nuts, 54
    and omega-3 fatty acids,
        50
sulforaphane, 40, 95
sulfur compounds, 9
    and beans, 55
    and spirulina, 74
    See also thiols.
sunflower seeds, 33, 52
    fat makeup of, 53
superoxide, 37

Surgeon General's Report
    on Nutrition and
    Health (1988), 27
Swiss chard, 19, 47
swordfish, 33, 36, 51

T-cells (T-lymphocytes), 32
    and mushrooms, 62
tangerines, 9, 36
    and immunity, 33
tannins, 60
Taylor, Philip R., 18–20
tea, 33, 60, 63–64
    black, 63–64, 68
    green, 27, 64
    oolong, 68
tempeh, 10, 42
    Red Pepper Tempeh, 107
    Tempeh with Garlic
        Sauce, 109
    Tempeh with Pine Nuts
        and Morels, 112
terpenoids, 9, 40, 46, 75, 125
    and cancer, 46
    sources of, 200
    types of, 9
thiamin. *See* vitamin B₁.
thioallyls, 29, 39
thiols, 9
    sources of, 199
    See also sulfer compounds.
Thomas Food Industry
    Register, 17
thrombosis, 58
tocopherol. *See* vitamin E.
tocotrienol. *See* vitamin E.
tofu, 10, 12
    Cilantro–Walnut Tofu, 110
    Spicy Tofu Dal, 105
    Spicy Tofu Steaks, 111
tomato(es), 2, 20, 25, 29,
    36, 40–41
    canned, 83
    Cilantro Salsa, 94
    and gamma linolenic acid,
        65

Hot Gingered Tomatoes,
    94
and immunity, 33
juice, 19
paste, 19
phytochemicals in, 86
raw, 19
San Francisco Cioppino,
    87
Sherried Tomato Bisque,
    89
Sicilian Tomato Salad, 88
Spanish Paella, 93
Spicy Stuffed Tomatoes,
    91
Tomato–Bean Salad with
    Parsley, 88
Veggie Medley Tomato
    Sauce, 90
Wild Mushroom
    Calzones, 92
triglycerides, 30, 50
triticale, 27, 45
trout (rainbow), 51
Tufts University, 46
tuna, 24, 51
    and immunity, 33
turmeric, 27, 67–68
turnip greens, 47

U.S. Food and Drug
    Administration (FDA),
    1–2
ubiquinone, 77
ultraviolet radiation, 25
University of California at
    Berkeley, 25, 34
University of North
    Carolina School of
    Medicine at Chapel
    Hill, 19, 21, 28–29
urinary-tract infections, 48,
    67
    and bilberry, 71

Vaccinium myrtilus, 71

varicose veins, 49

vasodilatation, 50

vegetables, 17, 25, 26, 27, 29, 33, 35

   Asparagus with Ginger–Orange Glaze, 128

   and cancer, 58

   Collard and Carrot Raita, 138

   cruciferous, 2, 10, 27, 39, 40, 41–42

      Broccoli–Cauliflower Bisque, 100

      Broccoli and Pine-Nut Casserole, 96

      Broccoli Rabe Stir-Fry, 102

      Brussels Sprouts with Honey–Ginger Glaze, 98

      Cauliflower Paratha, 99

      Indian Vegetable Curry, 97

      Peppered Cabbage Stew, 103

      phytochemicals in, 95

      Red and Green Cabbage Salad, 100

      Smoky Shiitake–Brussels Sprouts Salad, 98

      Wild Mushroom Cabbage Rolls, 101

   and ellagic acid, 54

   and fiber, 49, 58

   red/orange/yellow, 49–50

      Baked Kale with Parsnips and Carrots, 141

      Beets and Field Greens with Walnuts, 157

      Carrot–Coconut Bisque, 155

      Curried Yam Soup, 159

      Garlic Hummus with Roasted Red Peppers, 192

      Garlic-Stuffed Red Peppers, 191

      Hearty Pumpkin Soup with Pepitas, 154

      Millet and Summer Squash Casserole, 119

      Orange Pepper Champagne Glaze, 159

      phytochemicals in, 152

      Roasted Red Pepper Sauce, 156

      Salmon Paté with Roasted Red Pepper and Chives, 161

      Sautéed Peppers on Braised Radicchio, 157

      Spicy Sweet Potato Unfries, 156

      Stuffed Red Peppers with Basil–Basmati Rice, 158

      Sweet and Spicy Carrot Salad, 153

   Seven-Vegetable Pasta with Tarragon Glaze, 117

   Veggie Medley Tomato Sauce, 90

vegetarianism, 12

violaxanthins, 74

vitamin A, 6, 9, 17, 20, 24, 38, 40, 143

   and beans, 55

   best food sources of, 36

   and cancer, 25–26, 50

   and cruciferous vegetables, 40, 41, 95

   and greens, 47, 134

   and infections, 32

   precursors, 9

   and red/orange/yellow vegetables, 49, 152

   and tomatoes, 40, 86

   toxicity, 20

   and zoochemicals, 160

vitamin B. *See* B vitamins

vitamin B_1, 35

vitamin B_2, 35

vitamin B_3, 20

vitamin B_5, 38

vitamin B_6, 20

vitamin B_{12}, 38

Vitamin Book, The, 35, 47

vitamin C, 1, 2, 6, 9, 14, 17, 24, 38, 40

   and alfalfa, 74

   and barley grass, 73

   best food sources of, 36

   and cancer, 25, 26–27

   and cardiovascular disease, 29

   cereal grasses, 72

   and citrus, 46, 125

   and fruit, 49, 143

   and cruciferous vegetables, 40, 41, 95

   and greens, 47, 134

   and hypertension, 31

   and immunity, 32–33

   and isoflavones, 54

   and nitrosamines, 26

   and scurvy, 1, 12, 16, 45

   sources of, 200

   and tomatoes, 40, 86

   and red/orange/yellow vegetables, 49, 152

vitamin D, 21

vitamin E, 2, 6, 9, 14, 15, 16, 21, 24, 38, 40, 43, 45

   and Alzheimer's disease, 35

   and barley grass, 73

   best food sources of, 36

   and cancer, 26, 43

   and cardiovascular disease, 28, 43

   and co-Q 10, 77, 78, 79

   and fish oils, 51

   and free radicals, 34–35

   and immunity, 32, 33, 43

   and nitrosamines, 26

   and nuts, 54, 170

   and Parkinson's disease, 35

   and seeds, 54, 170

   sources of, 200

   toxicity, 20

and turmeric, 67
and whole grains, 43, 45,
    114. *See also* isoprenoids.
vitamin H. *See* biotin.
vitamins, 2, 8

Wall Street Journal, The, 25
walnuts, 33, 35, 52, 53
watercress, 19, 36, 47
    and immunity, 33
watermelon, 19, 48
    and immunity, 33
wheat germ, 28, 35, 37
    and immunity, 33

wheat, 27, 28, 43
    berries, 85
    bulgur, 44
        cooking time, 85
    grass, 73
    types of, 45
whitefish, 36
whooping cough, 14
Wigmore, Ann, 73
wine (red), 60–61
World Health Organiza-
    tion, 44

xanthophylls, 74, 75

yams, 33, 49
yogurt, 14

zeaxanthin, 18–19, 48, 143,
    152. *See also* carotenoids.
Zimmerman, Marcia, 9
zinc, 2, 38
    and immune function, 2,
        33
zoochemicals, x–xi, 2
    definition of, 7
    and fish, 160
zoonutrients, 7. *See also*
    zoochemicals.

INDEX

235